Contents

Acknowledgments

Thank you, Robert, for your unfailing support and love during my writing projects. Thank you William, Nicole, and Ericka. A special thanks to the contributing authors: Jay R. Lucker, Ronald C. Pearlman, and Wilhelmina Wright-Harp. To my graduate students: A good clinician is one who knows all of the latest approaches to patient management; an excellent clinician is one who listens with both the heart and the head.

Supporting Family Caregivers of Adults With Communication Disorders

A Resource Guide for Speech-Language Pathologists and Audiologists

Joan C. Payne, PhD

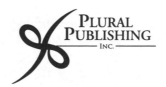

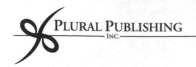

5521 Ruffin Road
San Diego, CA 92123

e-mail: info@pluralpublishing.com
Web site: http://www.pluralpublishing.com

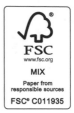

FSC
www.fsc.org
MIX
Paper from
responsible sources
FSC® C011935

Copyright © by Plural Publishing, Inc. 2015

Typeset in 11/13 Garamond by Flanagan's Publishing Services, Inc.
Printed in the United States of America by McNaughton & Gunn, Inc.

All rights, including that of translation, reserved. No part of this publication
may be reproduced, stored in a retrieval system, or transmitted in any form
or by any means, electronic, mechanical, recording, or otherwise, including
photocopying, recording, taping, Web distribution, or information storage
and retrieval systems without the prior written consent of the publisher.

For permission to use material from this text, contact us by
Telephone: (866) 758-7251
Fax: (888) 758-7255
e-mail: permissions@pluralpublishing.com

*Every attempt has been made to contact the copyright holders for material
originally printed in another source. If any have been inadvertently overlooked, the publishers will gladly make the necessary arrangements at the
first opportunity.*

Library of Congress Cataloging-in-Publication Data

Payne, Joan C., author.
  Supporting family caregivers of adults with communication disorders : a
resource guide for speech-language pathologists and audiologists / Joan C.
Payne.
        p. ; cm.
  Includes bibliographical references and index.
  ISBN 978-1-59756-502-8 (alk. paper) — ISBN 1-59756-502-4 (alk. paper)
  I. Title.
  [DNLM: 1. Caregivers. 2. Communication Disorders—psychology. 3. Adult.
4. Communication Disorders—nursing. WL 340.2]
  RC428.8
  616.85'50651—dc23
                                                       2015003271

Contributors

Jay R. Lucker, EdD, CCC-A/SLP, FAAA
Associate Professor
Department of Communication Sciences and Disorders
Howard University
Washington, DC
Chapter 5

Joan C. Payne, PhD
Professor and Interim Chair
Department of Communication Sciences and Disorders
School of Communications
Howard University
Washington, DC
Chapters 1, 2, 3, 4, 5, 6, 7, and 9

Ronald C. Pearlman, PhD, CCC-A, FAAA
Professor of Audiology
Department of Communication Sciences and Disorders
Howard University
Washington, DC
Chapter 5

Wilhelmina Wright-Harp, PhD, CCC-SLP, ASHA Fellow
Associate Dean of Research and Academic Affairs
Associate Professor
School of Communications
Howard University
Washington, DC
Chapter 8

This book is dedicated to two very independent, beautiful, and feisty ladies: the late Dr. Gretchen B. Payne and Mrs. Evelyn Bradley. Thank you both for allowing me to be your caregiver and walk with you on this journey called life. I am the better person for our experiences together.

1

Introduction

Joan C. Payne

Family caregivers, also called informal caregivers as opposed to those who are paid to render care, are vital extensions of the health care system. Without them, many persons discharged from acute and rehabilitative hospitals would not be able to care for themselves. The efforts of family caregivers are so important to the health, positive mental outlook, and indeed, survival of care recipients that their services are invaluable and predicted to be needed more and more as the 21st century continues.

This book is designed to provide information on the roles, obligations, stressors, and cultural dynamics of caregiving, as well as instruments for measuring caregiver reactions to caring responsibilities, referral sources, and resource information. The purpose of putting this information in one place where it is readily accessible is to empower speech-language pathologists and audiologists to support family caregivers of adults with disorders of communication and swallowing.

Caregiving is a deeply personal and intensive enterprise. Many caregivers report that they have appreciated the time to develop more intimate and caring relationships with their loved ones. Their joy, they say, is in giving back to others with whom they have forged significant bonds or who were once their caregivers, including parents, siblings, grandparents, uncles, aunts, in-laws, and family friends.

At the same time, a significant body of research indicates that caregiving is also costly in terms of time, effort, and financial sacrifices. Many caregivers are placed in the primary role of helping others without adequate resources with which to provide the best care. Caregiving can be so stressful that caregivers can themselves develop diseases and disabling conditions that affect their caregiving and those who depend on them. For some, the stress can be so crippling that some caregivers are forced to abandon providing care altogether, or they become terminally ill.

Speech-language pathologists and audiologists recognize the commitment and contributions of family caregivers. Several researchers have already begun to document the roles and needs of family caregivers in the literature on aphasia and stroke (Rombough, Howse, & Bartfay, 2006); end-of-life decisions (Williams & Harvey, 2013); professionals' support of family caregivers (Payne, 2009); dysphagia (Leslie, Miller, & Redle, 2011); and, training formal (paid) caregivers to work with dementia patients (Wilson, Rochon, Milhailidis, & Leonard, 2012). The American Speech-Language-Hearing Association's (ASHA) website of resources for stroke patients and their families has been hailed as an important and needed resource (ASHA, 2013). More needs to be done, however. Speech-language pathologists and audiologists need a toolkit of information and resources to educate and assist family caregivers. That is the intent of this resource guide.

To that end, Chapter 2 gives an overview of statistics on family caregivers, caregiver responsibilities for care, the economics of family caregiving, and concepts of caregiver burden, strain, and stress. In addition, information on the effects of caregiving on the physical, mental, and emotional health of those who provide care is also provided. Caregiving has been recognized as an important national resource. There are laws that protect and support caregivers at the local and national levels, and Chapter 2 also includes national and state legislation that supports family caregivers while they deliver care.

Chapter 3 describes the diversity of caregivers and how culture and tradition prescribe who will care for disabled adults as well as how caregivers use both internal and external resources. There are important differences in how caregivers perceive and accept caregiving responsibilities across ethnic and cultural groups. These differences have implications for how caregivers manage when the responsibilities become stressful. There are also some differences in how caregivers may accept and comply with counseling and referrals. Speech-language pathologists and audiologists will need to consider these differences in order to provide the most culturally competent assistance.

Chapter 4 discusses basic characteristics of various brain-based diseases and disorders that affect communication and swallowing with a focus on how these disabling conditions affect caregivers. Recommendations are given to enable speech-language pathologists to help caregivers to work with adults who have communication and swallowing disorders and to assist them to minimize communication breakdowns.

Chapter 5 is developed from the perspective of audiologists and includes basic information on hearing loss, auditory processing disorders, balance disorders, cochlear implants and hearing aids, as well as the impact on caregivers. Included in this chapter is information on helping caregivers to maintain hearing aids and cochlear implants in good working order. A major portion of the chapter is devoted to providing information about assistive and augmentative technologies which audiologists can use to educate caregivers of adults with hearing loss about who can benefit from these devices.

Perceptions of burden, strain, and stress interfere with a caregiver's ability to provide quality and sustained care. Chapter 6 describes assessments that measure caregiver strain, burden, stress, and coping with caring responsibilities. A variety of measures are included that are used by health professionals to assess how caregivers are functioning in their roles. These are provided to acquaint speech-language pathologists and audiologists with the available measures and their purposes. Some assessments measure caregiver burden, and others measure stress, strain, or coping. One tool, a measure of coping, is specifically mentioned as a possible instrument that can be used with caregivers of adults with communication or swallowing disorders.

Chapter 7 introduces concepts of education and counseling caregivers within the clinical setting and within the scope of practice. Educating and training caregivers can be helpful in improving communication and providing a continuum of therapy outside of the clinical setting. Although speech-language pathologists and audiologists do not provide counseling in many areas of need, resource information is provided that can be shared with caregivers which will empower them to find answers to their most important questions, like respite or hospice care, elder law, and insurance.

Chapter 8 provides information on other health care professionals and their areas of expertise. It is designed to inform speech-language pathologists and audiologists about the most appropriate professionals to whom caregivers should be referred when they need counseling in specific areas outside of the scope of practice.

Chapter 9 concludes with a case presentation and questions for clinicians to answer about how caregivers can be supported.

It is hoped that this book will serve as a resource for professionals and students in speech-language pathology and audiology and a part of the toolkit for assisting caregivers. It is also the intent that this resource book will be helpful to those who are involved in caregiving now and in the future. Perhaps former First Lady Rosalyne Carter said it best:

> There are only four kinds of people in the world—
> Those who have been caregivers;
> Those who are currently caregivers;
> Those who will be caregivers; and,
> Those who will need caregivers.

References

American Speech-Language-Hearing Association. (2013). *ASHA stroke page highly ranked as caregiver resource site rated among the best of its kind*. Retrieved from http://www.asha.org/About/news/Press-Releases/2013/ASHA-Caregiver-Resource.htm#sthash.JRSKRU4S.dpuf

Leslie, P., Miller, A., & Redle, E. (2011). *Caregiver burden across the lifespan*. Presentation at the 2011 Convention of the American Speech-Language-Hearing Association, San Diego, CA.

Payne, J. C. (2009, March 3). Supporting family caregivers: The role of speech-language pathologists and audiologists. *The ASHA Leader*. Retrieved from http://www.asha.org/publications/leader/2009/090 303/090303d/

Rombough, R. E., Howse, E. L., & Bartfay, W. J. (2006). Caregiver strain and caregiver burden of primary caregivers of stroke survivors with and without aphasia. *Rehabilitation Nursing, 31*, 199–209.

Williams, S. W., & Harvey, I. S. (2013). Culture, race, and SES: Application to end of life decision making for African American caregivers. *Perspectives on Gerontology, 18*, 69–76. Retrieved from http://sig15 perspectives.pubs.asha.org/article.aspx?articleid=1813576

Wilson, R., Rochon, E., Mihailidis, A., & Leonard, C. (2012). Examining success of communication strategies used by formal caregivers assisting individuals with Alzheimer's disease during an activity of daily living. *Journal of Speech, Language, and Hearing Research, 55*, 328–341. doi:10.1044/1092-4388(2011/10-0206)

2

The Dynamics of Family Caregiving

Joan C. Payne

Who Are Family Caregivers?

Family caregivers are major contributors to the quality of life and wellness of persons in their care, and essential to the success of any health-related intervention program. Within the United States, a significant number of persons are designated as family caregivers. State-by-state analyses show that there are millions of family caregivers who are providing continuous support to adults who can no longer care for themselves (National Alliance for Caregiving in collaboration with AARP, 2009).

As of 2009, 65.7 million caregivers make up 29% of the U.S. adult population providing care to someone who is ill, disabled, or aged (National Alliance for Caregiving in collaboration with AARP, 2009). An estimated 52 million caregivers provide care to adults over age 18 with a disability or illness (Coughlin, 2010). In addition, 43.5 million adult family caregivers care for someone aged 50 years and older, and 14.9 million care for someone who has Alzheimer's disease or other dementias (Alzheimer's Association, 2011). Caregivers who help an older adult say that the main problem or illness the person they care for has is aging (15%) followed by diabetes, cancer, and heart disease. One quarter (25%) of caregivers helping an older adult report that the person they care for is suffering from Alzheimer's disease, another type of dementia, or other mental confusion, but less than one in ten (8%) say this is their care recipient's main problem or illness (Alzheimer's Association, 2011).

Previous descriptions of the impact of family caregiving on society suggest that family support is a buffer to stress and provides positive outcomes for family members (Reinhard, Given, Petlick, & Bemis, 2008). Earlier, Cantor (1991) proposed a social care model of kinship support that has relevance for present-day consideration. According to Cantor, there are three major areas of kin and non-kin assistance: socialization and self-actualization, instrumental tasks of daily living, and personal care assistance in time of illness or crises. In his view, older adults tend to rely most heavily on spouses and adult children for instrumental, task-oriented support; their friends and spouses (usually the husband) for confiding support; and their groups, organizations, and acquaintances for esteem support.

The prevailing thought is that the quality and variety of supportive relationships decrease the number of health risks that cause or exacerbate major illness. Support networks also function to sustain older adults in time of changing health status. Overall, families are the major societal mechanism for the production of positive outcomes for their members (Brown, 1990; Feinberg, 2013).

How Is Family Caregiving Provided?

Family caregivers provide unpaid assistance for 20 hours or more weekly for the physical and emotional needs of another person. Another definition is that a family caregiver is someone over the age of 18 years old who has provided unpaid care to a relative or friend over the age of 18 years old in the last 12 months

(National Alliance for Caregiving & Evercare, 2006). In order to appreciate the roles and responsibilities of family caregivers, it is necessary to clarify who in an individual's support network provides the most intense level of care. Increasingly, once a person is discharged from acute care, hands-on care, generally in a home, is provided by family and friends. The home may be that of the caregiver or the care recipient. Many family caregivers care for a loved one from a long-distance location. Family caregivers also advocate for persons in the institutional setting. Those who provide care of this type are called family caregivers (Family Caregiver Alliance, 2014). The acceptance of caregiving responsibilities has its foundation in a relationship, but the act of caregiving is an additional role that requires preparation, acceptance, support, and resources (Reinhard, Feinberg, & Choula, 2011).

What Is Meant by "Family"?

Family refers to persons who share a profound and loving relationship with one another. Hence, the designation of family includes those with whom a caregiver is related by blood, such as children, siblings, aunts, uncles, and grandparents, and also includes stepparents, in-law parents and grandparents, spouses, and domestic partners (U.S. Department of Labor, 2014). Friends and fictive kin also provide caregiving. Fictive kin are persons who are regarded as close as family, such as "Play Mother," and who assume in many ways the roles of persons related by blood (Payne, 1992). Approximately 83% of 1,247 caregivers interviewed reported that they are caring for relatives while 17% reported caring for people outside of the family (National Alliance for Caregiving in collaboration with AARP, 2004).

Although caregiving is often described as loving and rewarding, there is consensus that caregiving can be stressful for both the caregiver and the care recipient. Fear of the unknown, fear that resources are not adequate, anxiety about health problems, and grief for the inevitable changes caused by diseases and disorders can affect quality of life for the entire support network as well as for the patient. Density and quality of friend and family supports can serve to decrease the level of anxiety in persons who are receiving care.

Responsibilities of Family Caregivers

Caregiving lasts an average of 4.6 years (National Alliance for Caregiving in collaboration with AARP, 2009). Family caregivers provide care, ranging from partial assistance to 24-hour care, depending on the severity of the disease, disorder, or condition. Most family caregivers report that they provide unpaid care to chronically ill or disabled older persons for 20 hours a week or more and donate physical, instrumental (help with daily living tasks), emotional, psychological, and often financial assistance to those who are in their care.

Assistance in activities of daily living (ADLs) means that the caregiver provides those services that maintain the individual's health and well-being at the most rudimentary and critical levels, such as assisting limited or nonambulatory care recipients with transference, toileting, bathing, and other personal hygiene needs, feeding (if needed), and ensuring that medicine is taken. Help with instrumental activities of daily living (IADLs) includes providing assistance in such activities as food preparation, shopping, running errands, paying bills, providing transportation, and meeting with medical and rehabilitative personnel on behalf of the care recipient (National Alliance for Caregiving in collaboration with AARP, 2009).

Results of the Home Alone study (AARP with United Health Hospital Fund, 2012) clearly show how challenging caregiver tasks are when there is a need to provide complex chronic care. Nearly half of the caregivers surveyed (46% or 777) performed medical and nursing tasks. More than 96% (747) also provided ADL supports (e.g., personal hygiene, dressing/undressing, or getting in and out of bed) or IADL support (e.g., taking prescribed medications, shopping for groceries, transportation, or using technology) or both. Of these caregivers nearly two-thirds (501) reported that they did all three types of tasks. Of the nonmedical family caregivers, two-thirds (605) provided IADL assistance only (AARP with United Health Hospital Fund, 2012; Reinhard, Levine, & Samis, 2012).

Family caregivers also provide more intangible types of care such as psychological, spiritual, and emotional support. The close relationship between the caregiver and care recipient is a shared relationship with involved emotions, experiences, and memories (Alzheimer's Association, 2011). This type of support bolsters self-confidence, helps the care recipient to adjust to restrictions brought on by disabling conditions, facilitates acceptance of new physical realities and self-image, and/or prepares the care recipient for the end of life.

Caregiver Roles

Caregivers tend to function in primary or secondary roles (Keith, 1995). Primary caregivers are those who bear the heaviest responsibility for daily care, while secondary care providers, often other relatives and friends who function as partners or within teams, provide more limited support. Although men are increasingly functioning as primary family caregivers, the typical primary family caregiver is a mature (average age is 48 years), working woman who is providing 20 hours or more of unpaid care for an aging parent, usually her mother. Hence, the term, "sandwich generation" speaks to the difficulties often experienced by women caregivers who find themselves caring for an ill family member, sometimes from a long distance, while still working and often parenting children or young adults.

Children and young adults between 8 and 18 years of age participate actively in family caregiving as well, although most are not the sole providers. There are an estimated 1.3 to 1.4 million child caregivers nationally. Child caregivers tend to live in households with lower incomes than do noncaregivers. Most are caring for a parent or a grandparent and are less likely to live in two-parent households. Alzheimer's disease is the most common care recipient's condition (National Alliance for Caregiving & the United Hospital Fund, 2005).

Psychological and emotional support are also part of the secondary caregiver's role. Secondary caregivers, often other relatives and friends, often assist the primary caregiver by providing help with physical and emotional care or by providing respite for the primary caregiver.

Gender Differences in Caregiving

An estimated 66% of caregivers are female. One-third (34%) take care of two or more people (National Alliance for Caregiving in collaboration with AARP, 2009). However, approximately one-third of the nation's caregivers are men, although they do not report the highest level(s) of caregiver burden (National Alliance for Caregiving in collaboration with AARP, 2004). The gender balance shifts to close to equal participation between men and women among spousal caregivers aged 75 years and older (McCann et al., 2000) and for those caring for 18- to 49-year-old care recipients (47% of caregivers are male). However, more women than men (32% male, 68% female) care for persons over the age of 50 (National Alliance for Caregiving in collaboration with AARP, 2009).

The number of male caregivers may be increasing and will continue to do so due to a variety of social demographic factors such as divorce (Kramer, 2002). Male caregivers tend to help other men while female caregivers help fewer men. That is, about one in three (35%) male caregivers help male care recipients, whereas only 28% of female caregivers help male care recipients. Male caregivers are more likely to be working full or part time than female caregivers (National Alliance for Caregiving in collaboration with AARP, 2009).

Women provide the majority of formal and informal care to spouses, parents, parents-in-law, friends, and neighbors, and they play many roles while caregiving—hands-on health provider, care manager, friend, companion, surrogate decision maker, and advocate. Overall, female caregivers provide more hours of care and a higher level of care than male caregivers. For example, women spend an average of four hours more caregiving per week than men and are also more likely to say they feel they did not have a choice in taking on this role than men (National Alliance for Caregiving in collaboration with AARP, 2004). Women are more likely, also, to engage in hands-on support for the more ill or disabled friends or family members, whereas men respond to loved one's needs for support by delaying retirement, in part to shoulder the financial burden associated with long-term care (National Alliance for Caregiving in collaboration with AARP, 2009).

Burden of Care

Three definitions serve to illustrate the effect of caregiving on those who provide care. *Caregiver burden* is defined as the emotional, physical, and financial demands and responsibilities of an individual's illness that are placed on family members, friends, or other individuals involved with the individual outside the health care system. *Caregiver burden* has also been defined as the strain or load borne by a person who cares for a chronically ill, disabled, or elderly family member (Stucki & Mulvey, 2000). *Caregiver strain* occurs when the caregiver perceives that he or she has difficulty in performing the responsibilities of caregiving (Buhse, 2008). *Caregiver stress* is a result of the emotional and physical strain of caregiving. It can take many forms. For instance, the caregiver may feel

- frustrated and angry about taking care of someone with dementia who often wanders away or becomes easily upset;
- guilty, out of the anxiety that he or she should be able to provide better care, despite all the other responsibilities;
- lonely, because caregiving has limited an outside social life; and
- exhausted and sleep deprived.

Caregiver stress appears to affect women more than men. About 75% of caregivers who report feeling very strained emotionally, physically, or financially are women (Buhse, 2009).

The concept of the burden of care was defined in 1980 by Steven H. Zarit, an American gerontologist, to describe the discomfort experienced by the principal caregiver of an older family member, and the negative effects of caregiving on the caregiver's health, psychological well-being, finances, and social life (Zarit, Reever, & Bach-Peterson, 1980). Dimensions calculated for levels of care are amount of time spent and type of care, whether IADLs (e.g., housekeeping help, grocery shopping, managing finances or bills, preparing meals, arranging/supervising outside services or activities) or ADLs (e.g., bathing/showering, taking to the toilet, feeding, giving medications, dealing with incontinence or diapers, getting dressed, getting in or out of beds or chairs) (Kim & Shulz, 2008). The combination of time spent weekly and number of ADLs and IADLs provided determines the Level of Burden Index, which is a 1 to 5 scale, with 1 meaning the least caregiver responsibility, and 5 designating the greatest amount of responsibility. The degree of burden is calculated from answers to the 22-item *Burden Interview* (Zarit, Reevers, & Bach-Peterson, 1980) found in Table 2–1.

The level of care that caregivers say they provide has an impact on the caregiver's load. Based upon interviews with over 1,200 caregivers (National Alliance for Caregiving in collaboration with AARP, 2004), half of all caregivers (50%) aged 18 and older say they provide care at the lower ranges of the Level of Burden Index (33% at Level 1 and 17% at Level 2). A nearly equal percentage of caregivers report that they are the middle of the index (15%) or that they provide care at the higher ranges of the index (31%). This measurement of levels is important because indices of Level of Burden (i.e., having a choice to take on caregiving responsibilities and caregivers' reported health status) appear to have the greatest influence on whether caregivers perceive emotional stress, physical strain, or financial hardship as a result of being a caregiver.

Perceptions of level of burden are also influenced by the type and severity of the disability of the care recipient. Kim and Schulz (2008) compared levels of burden for care recipients with dementia, cancer, diabetes, or frailty, and found that dementia and cancer care were reported by caregivers to be the two most burdensome care responsibilities, followed by care recipients with diabetes and lastly, the frail elderly. Although caregiver stress in caring for persons with dementia has been well documented, much less has been written about the stressors of caring for persons with cancer. This suggests that more support for caregivers of persons with cancer is warranted (Kim & Schulz, 2008).

Table 2–1. The Burden Interview

Instructions	The Burden Interview has been specially designed to reflect the stresses experienced by caregivers of dementia patients. It can be completed by caregivers themselves or as part of an interview. Caregivers are asked to respond to a series of 22 questions about the impact of the patient's disabilities on their life. For each item, caregivers are to indicate how often they felt that way (never, rarely, sometimes, quite frequently, or nearly always).
Scoring	The Burden Interview is scored by adding the numbered responses of the individual items. Higher scores indicate greater caregiver distress. The Burden Interview, however, should not be taken as the only indicator of the caregiver's emotional state. Clinical observations and other instruments, such as measures of depression, should be used to supplement this measure. Norms for the Burden Interview have not been computed, but estimates of the degree of burden can be made from preliminary findings. These are: 0–20, little or no burden; 21–40, mild to moderate burden; 41–60, moderate to severe burden; and 61–88, severe burden.

The following is a list of statements which reflect how people sometimes feel when taking care of another person. After each statement, indicate how often you feel that way: (0) never, (1) rarely, (2) sometimes, (3) quite frequently, or (4) nearly always. There are no right or wrong answers.

1. Do you feel that your relative asks for more help than he or she needs?   0   1   2   3   4

2. Do you feel that, because of the time you spend with your relative, you don't have enough time for yourself?   0   1   2   3   4

3. Do you feel stressed between caring for your relative and trying to meet other responsibilities for your family or work?   0   1   2   3   4

4. Do you feel embarrassed about your relative's behavior?   0   1   2   3   4

5. Do you feel angry when you are around your relative?   0   1   2   3   4

6. Do you feel that your relative currently affects your relationship with other family members?   0   1   2   3   4

continues

Table 2–1. *continued*

7.	Are you afraid about what the future holds for your relative?	0	1	2	3	4
8.	Do you feel that your relative is dependent upon you?	0	1	2	3	4
9.	Do you feel strained when you are around your relative?	0	1	2	3	4
10.	Do you feel that your health has suffered because of your involvement with your relative?	0	1	2	3	4
11.	Do you feel that you don't have as much privacy as you would like, because of your relative?	0	1	2	3	4
12.	Do you feel that your social life has suffered because you are caring for your relative?	0	1	2	3	4
13.	Do you feel uncomfortable having your friends over because of your relative?	0	1	2	3	4
14.	Do you feel that your relative seems to expect you to take care of him or her, as if you were the only one he or she could depend on?	0	1	2	3	4
15.	Do you feel that you don't have enough money to care for your relative, in addition to the rest of your expenses?	0	1	2	3	4
16.	Do you feel that you will be unable to take care of your relative much longer?	0	1	2	3	4
17.	Do you feel that you have lost control of your life since your relative's death?	0	1	2	3	4
18.	Do you wish that you could just leave the care of your relative to someone else?	0	1	2	3	4
19.	Do you feel uncertain about what to do about your relative?	0	1	2	3	4
20.	Do you feel that you should be doing more for your relative?	0	1	2	3	4
21.	Do you feel that you could do a better job in caring for your relative?	0	1	2	3	4
22.	Overall, how burdened do you feel in caring for your relative?	0	1	2	3	4

Source: Zarit, S. H., Reever, K. E., & Bach-Peterson. (1980). Relatives of the impaired elderly: Correlates of feelings of burden. *The Gerontologist, 20,* 649–655. Retrieved from https://www.healthcare.uiowa.edu/igec/tools/caregivers/burdenInterview.pdf

Effects of Caregiving on the Caregiver

Speech-language pathologists and audiologists can learn a great deal about the physical and emotional status of caregivers by listening and observing. For many caregivers, the benefits of caregiving far outweigh the stressors. However, some well-documented signs that a caregiver may be negatively affected by the responsibilities of providing continuous care are discussed below.

Effects on Physical Health

The process of caring can be so time consuming that some caregivers fail to keep regular medical and dental appointments, fail to get adequate rest and exercise, eat irregularly and poorly, and lose touch with their kinship, friendship, and spiritual supports. Low-income caregivers have an additional financial strain in caregiving which brings about considerable anxiety. These caregivers are more likely to report that their health is poor. Although most caregivers are in good health, it is not uncommon for caregivers to have serious health problems (Reinhard, Given, Petlick, & Beamis, 2008). It has been found, for example, that caregivers

- are more likely to be have symptoms of depression or anxiety;
- are more likely to have a long-term medical problem, such as heart disease, cancer, diabetes, or arthritis;
- have higher levels of stress hormones;
- spend more days sick with an infectious disease;
- have a weaker immune response to the influenza, or flu, vaccine;
- have slower wound healing;
- have higher levels of obesity; and,
- may be at higher risk for mental decline, including problems with memory and paying attention.

Additionally, many caregivers report that they simply do not feel healthy. Twenty-three percent (23%) of family caregivers caring for loved ones for five years or more report their health is fair or poor (National Alliance for Caregiving in collaboration with

AARP, 2009). Family caregivers are prone to having a chronic condition at more than twice the rate of noncaregivers. More than 1 in 10 (11%) family caregivers report that caregiving has caused their physical health to deteriorate (National Alliance for Caregiving & the United Hospital Fund, 2005).

The closer the family or kinship relationship, the more vulnerable caregivers may be. Similarly, the older the caregiver is, the more likely that the responsibilities of caregiving will have negative consequences on physical health. Elderly spousal caregivers, for example, with a history of chronic illness themselves and who are experiencing caregiving-related stress, have a significantly higher mortality rate than their noncaregiving peers. A wife's hospitalization increases her husband's chances of dying within a month by 35%. A husband's hospitalization boosts his wife's mortality risk by 44% (Census, 2005).

Extreme stress has a significant negative effect on health and can take as much as 10 years off a family caregiver's life. In particular, the stress of family caregiving for persons with dementia has been shown to impact a person's immune system for up to three years after their caregiving ends which increases their potential for developing a chronic illness (Kiecott-Glaser et al., 2003). Negative feelings of sadness, anger, and anxiety combined with the deleterious effects on health such as chronic illness and premature aging can take such a toll on caregivers that they may be physically unable to maintain a consistent level of support.

Effects on Emotional Health

Family caregivers who provide care 36 or more hours weekly are more likely than noncaregivers to experience symptoms of, depression or anxiety. For spouses, the rate is six times higher; for those caring for a parent the rate is twice as high (Glaser & Glaser, 2003; National Alliance for Caregiving in collaboration with AARP, 2009; National Alliance for Caregiving & Evercare, 2006).

Caregiver stress has a significant influence on one's ability to engage in the ongoing demands of family caregiving (Deeken, Taylor, Mangan, Yabroff, & Ingham, 2003) and is often the result of the caregiver feeling overly burdened in the role. Campbell and colleagues (2008) found that the strongest predictors of caregiver stress occurred when caregivers reported (a) a sense of "role captivity" or feelings of being trapped in their role as caregivers, (b) caregiver overload and fatigue, (c) adverse life events outside of the caregiving role, and (d) dissatisfaction with the relationship between caregiver and care recipient.

Caregiver stress also has a profound effect on the health and well-being of the person being cared for:

- Caregivers who have unmet needs or a high burden level may be impeded in their ability to be an ongoing support system for the disabled adult.
- Disabled adults are more likely to have unmet needs if their caregiver has a high degree of burden.
- A disabled adult's level of activity may decrease as his caregiver's psychological needs increase.
- Since a caregiver is a critical element of home care, if the burden on a caregiver becomes too great, the home care support may be seriously jeopardized.
- Increased caregiver burden increases the use of formal, paid helpers or an earlier institutionalization of the patient in a nursing home. (Deeken et al., 2003, p. 923)

Caregiver stress is frequently heightened by the care recipient's type and severity of illness. Han and Haley (1999) observed depression during both the acute and the chronic stages of stroke in their caregivers. Depression is a major indicator of caregiver burnout. Approximately 40% to 70% of family caregivers have clinically significant symptoms of depression with approximately a quarter to half of these caregivers meeting the diagnostic criteria for major depression (Zarit et al., 1980). Levels of psychological distress and stress are significantly higher, and levels of self-efficacy, subjective well-being, and physical health are significantly lower in dementia caregivers than in other caregivers (Brodaty & Donkin, 2009). Caregivers of dementia patients report more depression than those caring for a person with a physical disability.

Effects on Financial Stability

Research has shown that caregivers frequently must choose between working and caregiving and either reduce their working hours or quit working altogether, resulting in lost wages, benefits including insurance and retirement, and Social Security (Feinberg, Reinhard, Houser, & Choula, 2011; Houser & Gibson, 2008; Lai, 2012; Metropolitan Life Insurance Company, 1999).

Effects on Spousal and Family Relationships

Personal reports and research findings indicate that both spousal relationships, where a spouse is the caregiver, and family relationships often undergo change during the caregiving process. Spousal relationships are affected when a disabled spouse is no longer able to assume previous responsibilities, specifically, working, paying bills, doing household chores, or parenting. In many households, the other spouse must assume these tasks in addition to caregiving. Inability to communicate wants and needs also affects how spouses are able to interact with each other and marital conflicts are worsened by behavioral problems seen in such disorders as dementia (Ascher et al., 2010; DeVugt et al., 2006), cancer (Kim, Baker, Spiller, & Wellisch, 2006; Youngmee, Wellisch, & Spiller, 2008), stroke (Thompson & Ryan, 2009), and traumatic brain injuries (Kreutzer, Marwitz, & Kepler, 1992; Wood, Liossi, & Wood, 2005).

Positive change comes about when families unite to share in the caregiver burden. Family members report that they are drawn closer together and feel a sense of accomplishment when they work together to provide care. Negative change is reflected in caregivers' perception that they had no choice about assuming the work of caregiving or that their family members failed to share in the physical, emotional, or financial hardships of giving care. These feelings tend to persist long after the caregiving experience is over and color the ways in which families interact and support each other.

Caregiver Guilt and Grieving

Guilt is a consistent topic in the literature about caregiving. Caregiver guilt is, among other feelings, the sense that one has not done/is not doing enough to provide care. Among 739 caregivers of cancer patients, being young; caring for one's parents; working; stress; uncertainty about the ability to care properly; and poor mental, social, and physical functioning were significantly related with caregiver guilt (Spillers, Wellisch, Kim, Matthews, & Baker, 2008). Guilt was also associated with fatigue, stress, and loss of identity or a change of identity when adult children care for disabled parents or grandparents (Boquet, Oliver, Wittenberg-Lyles, Doorenbos, & Demiris, 2011) or when placing them in an institution (Whitlatch, Schur, Noelker, Ejaz, & Looman, 2001).

Grief is a common phenomenon in caregiving, whether it is from seeing a loved one change as a result of a chronic illness (called anticipatory grief) or from losing a loved one through death. Grieving is a deeply personal and complex process. Some feelings will be revisited as caregivers deal with their grief. According to the Family Caregiver Alliance (2014), grieving is an individual coping mechanism with several stages:

- Shock
- Emotional release
- Depression, loneliness, and a sense of isolation
- Physical symptoms of distress
- Feelings of panic
- A sense of guilt
- Anger or rage
- Inability to return to usual activities
- The gradual regaining of hope
- Acceptance as we adjust our lives to reality

Since guilt is an emotion that can affect how caregivers are able to provide care, clinicians should listen for indications that caregivers are troubled by guilt or indicate that they have unrealistic and negative opinions about their ability to provide care. Grief is a natural part of change in status or relationships. However, various somatic and emotional responses, such as sleeping too much, headaches, low energy or exhaustion, memory gaps, preoccupation, depression, and irritability are common complaints that can interfere with the caregiver's ability to provide care or to manage the daily routines of work and home. Caregivers are particularly vulnerable to illness while they are grieving, and it is important for them to give voice to their feelings as they go through the stages of grief (Family Caregivers Alliance, 2014). It is also important for caregivers to receive grief counseling from psychologists or pastoral counselors to cope with intense feelings of loss.

The Economics of Caregiving

Family caregivers will be needed increasingly to provide long-term complex care for disabled older adults. According to Feinberg and her colleagues (2011):

> The impact of shorter hospital stays, limited hospital discharge planning, and the spread of home-based medical technologies is reflected in the complex and physically demanding nursing tasks that family caregivers are increasingly carrying out in the home. They often have little training or preparation for performing these tasks, which include bandaging and wound care, tube feedings, managing catheters, giving injections, or operating medical equipment. Estimates of the proportion of family caregivers handling these health-related tasks in the home range from 23 percent to more than 53 percent. (p. 5)

Family caregiving is expensive, however. The value of unpaid family caregivers will likely continue to be the largest source of long-term care services in the United States because the aging population 65+ will more than double between the years 2000 and 2030, increasing to 71.5 million from 35.1 million in 2000 (Coughlin, 2010). Moreover, estimates of out-of-pocket expenses to caregivers caring for persons who are 50 years and older range from $4,570 for those caring for persons who live nearby, to $5,885 for caregivers whose care recipients live with them, to $8,728 for caregivers who provide long-distance care (Houser & Gibson, 2008).

The estimated annual cost of nursing home care is $50,000 per person, depending on where the care is located. About one-third of persons in care use their own resources to pay for their care, and a small percentage (5%) have long-term care insurance. Medicaid, a federal and state health insurance program for low-income persons, pays for care after all other personal savings have been exhausted. Medicare, the federal health insurance program for older persons and some younger persons with disability, pays for short-term nursing home stays (Feinberg, 2013; Feinberg et al., 2011).

Compared with nursing home costs, the estimated value of the services family caregivers provide for "free" was $450 billion a year in 2009 (Feinberg et al., 2011). That is almost twice as much as is actually spent on home care and nursing home services combined ($158 billion).

The recent economic downturn in the United States proved to be devastating for many family caregivers and posed financial challenges in lost wages from reduced work hours, time out of the workforce, family leave, or early retirement. More than one third of caregivers to persons aged 50 and older either quit their jobs or reduced their work hours. Currently, midlife women in the labor force who begin caregiving are more likely to quit working altogether (National Alliance for Caregiving in collaboration with AARP, 2009).

The caregiving time burden falls most heavily on lower-income women: 52% of women caregivers with incomes at or below the national median of $35,000 spend 20+ hours each week providing care (The Commonwealth Fund, 1999). For lower-income caregivers, accessing paid sources of care has been particularly difficult. In fact, lower-income caregivers are half as likely as higher-income caregivers to have paid home health care or assistance available to provide support for and relief from their caregiving functions. Increasingly, however, data from 2009 interviews suggest that some caregivers are using the Internet for caregiver help and are likely to request outside assistance (National Alliance for Caregiving in collaboration with AARP, 2009).

Key Legislation Affecting Caregivers and Disabled Adults

National Legislation

Caregivers may not be aware that there are national provisions to assist them in various ways. Table 2–2 gives four key laws that concern family caregivers of adults. One is the Affordable Care Act (ACA) that enables older adults to select affordable insurance from a marketplace of insurers and offers protections and benefits for seniors in the areas of preventive care, rehabilitation services, and costs for drugs. The ACA also provides for caregivers by

Table 2–2. Key Legislation Affecting Family Caregivers

Name of Legislation	Contact Agency
Affordable Care Act (ACA)	U.S. Department of Health and Human Services

New legislation (2010) has implications for caregivers of seniors with chronic, disabling conditions. The ACA was enacted to provide insurance options to more older adults, regardless of income. Older adults have the following protections under the Affordable Care Act as of 2014:

- The Act ends arbitrary withdrawals of insurance coverage and guarantees the right to appeal for reconsideration of denial of payment. The Act also ends lifetime limits on coverage for all new health insurance plans.
- Insurance companies, under the Act, must now publicly justify any unreasonable rate hikes. The Act protects the choice of doctors and covers preventive care at no cost, including vaccines.
- The Act removes insurance company barriers to emergency services at a hospital outside of the health plan's network and removes the insurance company's being able to deny payment because of pre-existing conditions.
- Eligible seniors who are in the Medicare coverage gap known as the "donut hole" automatically receive a discount on prescription drugs in 2011 and beyond.
- SLPs working with older patients at home must reassess each case by the 13th visit or every 30 days, whichever comes first, and perform a functional reassessment of the patient and compare the results to previous assessments. The purpose of this is to measure therapy effectiveness as treatment progresses.
- Seniors can secure insurance coverage in the Marketplace in the next open enrollment.

Caregiver supports are also addressed in the ACA in the following ways:

1. The law includes individuals and their caregivers as decision makers about care options, and it recognizes the need to address the caregiver's own experience of care in assessments and quality improvement of services.
2. The ACA promotes new models of care that identify the family caregiver as a key partner.
3. Third, it advances efforts to better prepare family caregivers to perform their care tasks.
4. Last, it enhances opportunities to expand home and community-based services (HCBS) and provide better support to caregiving families. The law explicitly mentions the term "caregiver" 46 times and "family caregiver" 11 times.

Table 2–2. *continued*

Sources:

http://www.hhs.gov/healthcare/insurance/index.html

Hasselkus, A. (2011). Working with older adults: Impact of the Affordable Care Act and other trends in health care. *Perspectives on Gerontology, 16*, 10–17. doi:10.1044/gero16.1.10

Feinberg, L., & Reamy, A. M. (2011). *Health reform law creates new opportunities to better recognize and support family caregivers.* Retrieved from http://assets .aarp.org/rgcenter/ppi/ltc/fs239.pdf

National Family Caregiver Support Program (NFCSP)   U.S. Administration on Aging

(OAA Title IIIE) Authorizing Legislation: Section 371 of the Older Americans Act (OAA) of 1965, as amended. The National Family Caregiver Support Program (NFCSP), established in 2000, provides grants to States and Territories, based on their share of the population aged 70 and over, to fund a range of supports that assist family and informal caregivers to care for their loved ones at home for as long as possible. The NFCSP offers a range of services to support family caregivers. Under this program, States shall provide five types of services:

- Information to caregivers about available services,
- Assistance to caregivers in gaining access to the services,
- Individual counseling, organization of support groups, and caregiver training,
- Respite care, and
- Supplemental services, on a limited basis.

Eligible program participants: Adult family members or other informal caregivers age 18 and older providing care to individuals 60 years of age and older; adult family members or other informal caregivers age 18 and older providing care to individuals of any age with Alzheimer's disease and related disorders.

Source: http://www.aoa.gov/aoa_programs/hcltc/caregiver/index.aspx

Caregivers and Veterans Omnibus Health Services Act of 2010 (Public Law 111-163)   Veteran's Administration

Under this law, family caregivers of veterans can receive:

- Training in providing personal care services to the veteran
- Ongoing technical support
- Counseling
- Lodging when accompanying the veteran to a Department facility

continues

Table 2–2. *continued*

The family caregiver who is the designated primary provider of personal care services to receive in addition:

- Mental health services
- Respite care not less than 30 days, including 24-hour per day care
- Medical care
- A monthly stipend

Source: American Psychological Association. Retrieved from http://www.apa.org/about/gr/issues/military/health-services-act.aspx

Family and Medical Leave Act of 1993 (FMLA)	**Department of Labor**

The FMLA entitles eligible employees of covered employers to take unpaid, job-protected leave for specified family and medical reasons with continuation of group health insurance coverage under the same terms and conditions as if the employee had not taken leave. Eligible employees are entitled to:

- Twelve workweeks of leave in a 12-month period for
  - the birth of a child and to care for the newborn child within one year of birth;
  - the placement with the employee of a child for adoption or foster care and to care for the newly placed child within one year of placement;
  - to care for the employee's spouse, child, or parent who has a serious health condition;
  - a serious health condition that makes the employee unable to perform the essential functions of his or her job;
  - any qualifying exigency arising out of the fact that the employee's spouse, son, daughter, or parent is a covered military member on "covered active duty"; or
  - Twenty-six workweeks of leave during a single 12-month period to care for a covered service member with a serious injury or illness if the eligible employee is the service member's spouse, son, daughter, parent, or next of kin (military caregiver leave).

Note: FMLA was amended in 2008 and the definition of family has been extended. Several states (California, Connecticut, Hawaii, Maine, Maryland, New Jersey, Rhode Island, Vermont, Wisconsin, and the District of Columbia) have their own definitions of family, including parents-in-law, grandparents, grandparents-in-law, step-parents, and domestic partners. It is being proposed to allow eligible employees in legal same-sex marriages to take FMLA leave to care for their spouse or family member, regardless of where they live. Also, there is a special eligibility for airline flight crew employees and an expansion of military family leave provisions.

Source: http://www.dol.gov/whd/fmla/

expanding services to them and by recognizing their role as decision makers. Next, the National Family Caregivers Support Program (NFCSP) funds supports to assist family caregivers to care for their loved ones at home for as long as possible. Another key legislation is the Caregivers and Veterans Omnibus Health Services Act of 2010 that provides support to caregivers of veterans. The fourth legislation is the Family and Medical Leave Act of 1993 (FMLA) that allows eligible employees to take a total of 12 workweeks of leave in a 12-month period to care for a family member with a serious health problem or a covered active duty military family member during exigent circumstances.

State Legislation

In 2003, 19 states had introduced or enacted legislation to assist caregivers. A list of those states and their legislation may be found on the National Alliance of Caregivers website (https://www.caregiver.org/archived-state-state-legislation).

The ACA is too new to assess the impact on caregivers and older adults. Provisions for adults rolled out only recently in 2014. The FMLA has helped eligible employees to be available to deliver up to 3 months of care without losing their jobs. The new definitions of family under the FMLA's state provisions recognize that the term "family" must be inclusive of the various ways that the concept family has expanded because of divorce, blended families, legislation regarding domestic partners, and gay marriages. Caregivers of veterans who were injured after 9/11 are eligible to apply to the Veterans Administration for a caregiving stipend. A report from the U.S. Department of Health and Human Services (n.d.) provides the following highlights about the NFCSP: In FY 2010, the most recent year for which service data are available, over 700,000 caregivers received services through the NFCSP. These services helped them better manage their caregiving responsibilities while ensuring their loved ones remained in the community for as long as possible. Service highlights include the following:

- *Access Assistance Services* provided over 1 million contacts to caregivers helping them locate services from a variety of private and voluntary agencies.

- *Counseling and Training Services* were provided over 125,000 caregivers with counseling, peer support groups, and training to help them better cope with the stresses of caregiving.
- *Respite Care Services* were provided more than 64,000 caregivers with 6.8 million hours with temporary relief—at home, or in an adult day care or institutional setting—from their caregiving responsibilities.

Data from AoA's national surveys of caregivers of elderly clients show the following:

- OAA services, including those provided through the NFCSP; are effective in helping caregivers keep their loved ones at home.
- Nearly 40% of caregivers report they have been providing care for 2 to 5 years while approximately 29% of family caregivers have been providing care for 5 to 10 years.
- It was found that 77% of caregivers of program clients report that services definitely enabled them to provide care longer than otherwise would have been possible.
- Approximately 89% of caregivers reported that services helped them to be better caregivers.
- Nearly half the caregivers of nursing-home-eligible care recipients indicated that the care recipient would be unable to remain at home without the support services.
- Nearly 12% of family caregivers reported they were caring for a grandson or granddaughter.

Future Projections

The numbers of family caregivers of adults are expected to increase dramatically over the next three decades. Current demographic projections predict a surge in the aging of America because of the Baby Boomers who are expected to live longer than the previous generation, survive what are generally considered to be catastrophic illnesses, and maintain themselves into old-old age, defined as age 85 and older. Veterans of wars in the Middle East are returning home with disabling injuries and will need continued family caregiving assistance.

The value of unpaid family caregivers will likely continue to be the largest source of long-term care services in the United States, and the aging population 65+ will more than double between the years 2000 and 2030 (The Commonwealth Fund, 1999), including injured veterans. A corollary to this is that many of these adults who are living longer will do so with chronic diseases and conditions that can lead to aphasia, swallowing disorders, sensorineural and balance disorders, auditory processing disturbances, progressive neurodegenerative motor diseases, and dementia. Each of these diseases and conditions or a combination of these disorders can disrupt hearing, speech, language, swallowing, and cognitive abilities significantly.

Regardless of the cause, when a person is unable to communicate, hear, or swallow normally, the burden of caregiving increases, and the dynamics in family relationships are profoundly affected. Loss of the ability to express one's needs and wants, the inability to obtain or give information, or simply to understand what is being said, or the injurious consequences of aspirating liquids or food, are perhaps the most devastating and frustrating consequences of poor health for both the caregiver and the care recipient.

Because of the multifaceted roles that family and informal caregivers play, they will need a range of supports to remain healthy, improve their caregiving skills, and remain in their caregiving role. Clinicians should be aware of the national and state laws that provide assistance and funding to caregivers or which protect working caregivers as they carry out their responsibilities. Many services are available through national and state government agencies, service organizations, faith-based organizations, and employers' assistance and leave programs.

Knowledge about and access to resources can serve to lessen depression, anxiety, and anger for many caregivers. Clinicians can assist caregivers by pointing out information about services and resources that support caregiving. Evidence shows that when caregivers receive support, they can delay nursing home placement or maintain the person in the home. For example, people with moderate dementia have been able to remain at home and defer nursing home placement by nearly 1.5 years when their family members receive counseling, information, and ongoing support (Family Caregiver Alliance, 2014).

As a result of functioning as members of management teams in acute care and rehabilitative care facilities, there are many opportunities for speech-language pathologists and audiologists to interact with family caregivers. As a part of assessment and intervention for the adult with communication disorders, speech-language pathologists and audiologists can be in pivotal positions to assist family caregivers (Payne, 2009).

Supporting family caregivers is good practice. Caregivers are invaluable resources for speech-language pathologists and audiologists. They are the best sources of information about a patient's functioning. Also, with professional guidance, caregivers can reinforce treatment goals in the home setting and can be instrumental in encouraging their care recipients to keep appointments and commitments to practice during and after therapy. Clinicians should keep in mind that although caregiving is rewarding, it is often accomplished at tremendous financial, physical, and emotional costs to caregivers. Caring for the caregiver, therefore, should be a priority in effective clinical management.

References

Alzheimer's Association. (2011). *Alzheimer's disease facts and figures*. Retrieved from http://www.alz.org/downloads/facts_figures_2011.pdf

American Association of Retired Persons (AARP) with the United Hospital Fund. (2012). *Home alone: Family caregivers providing complex chronic care*. Retrieved from http://www.aarp.org/content/dam/aarp/research/public_policy_institue/healh/home-alone-family-caregivers-providing-complex-chronic-care-revAARP-ppi-health.pdf

Ascher, E. A., Sturm, V. E., Seider, B. H., Holley, S. R., Miller, B. L. & Levenson, R. W. (2010). Relationship satisfaction and emotional language in frontotemporal dementia and Alzheimer disease patients and spousal caregivers. *Alzheimer's Disease and Associated Disorders*, *24*, 49–55. doi:10.1097/WAD.0b013e3181bd66a3

Boquet, J. R., Oliver, D. P., Wittenberg-Lyles, E., Doorenbos, A. Z., & Demiris, G. (2011). Taking care of a dying grandparent: Case studies of grandchildren in the hospice caregiver role. *Current Opinion in Psychiatry*, *16*, 629–633.

Brodaty, H., & Donkin, M. (2009). Family caregivers of people with dementia. *Dialogues in Clinical Neuroscience*, *11*, 217–228.

Brown, S. C. (1990). The prevalence of communicative disorders in the aging population. In E. Cherow (Ed.), *Proceedings of the research symposium on communication sciences and disorders and aging* (pp. 14–27). Rockville, MD: American Speech-Language-Hearing Association.

Buhse, M. (2008). Assessment of caregiver burden in families of persons with multiple sclerosis. *Journal of Neuroscience Nursing*, *40*, 25–31.

Campbell, P., Wright, J., Oyebode, J., Job, D., Crome, P., Bentham, P., . . . Lenden, C. (2008). Determinants of burden in those who care for someone with dementia. *International Journal of Geriatric Psychiatry*, *23*, 1078–1085.

Cantor, M. H. (1991). Neighbors and friends: An overlooked resource in the informal support system. *Research on Aging*, *1*, 434–463.

Census 2000 Special Report. (2005). *Disability and American families*. Retrieved from http://www.census.gov/prod/2005pubs/censr-23.pdf

Coughlin, J. (2010). *Estimating the impact of caregiving and employment on well-being: Outcomes and insights in health management* (Vol. 2, Issue 1). Retrieved from http://www.pascenter.org/publica tions/item.php?id=1092

Deeken, J. F., Taylor, K. L., Mangan, P., Yabroff, K. R., & Ingham, J. M. (2003). Care for the caregivers: A review of self-report instruments developed to measure the burden, needs, and quality of life of informal caregivers. *Journal of Pain and Symptom Management*, *26*, 922–953.

DeVugt, M. E., Riedijk, S. R., Aalten, P., Tibben, A., van Swieten, J. C., & Verhey, F. R. (2006). Impact of behavioral problems on spousal caregivers: A comparison between Alzheimer's disease and fronto-temporal dementia. *Dementia and Geriatric Cognitive Disorders*, *22*, 25–41.

Family Caregiver Alliance. (2014). *Caregiving*. Retrieved from https://www.caregiver.org/caregiving

Feinberg, L. (2013). *Keeping up with the times: Supporting family caregivers with workplace leave policies*. Washington, DC: AARP Public

Policy Institute. Retrieved from http://www.aarp.org/content/dam/aarp/research/public_policy_institute/ltc/2013/fmlainsight-keeping-up-with-time-AARP-ppi-ltc.pdf

Feinberg, L., Reinhard, S. C., Houser, A., & Choula, R. (2011). *Valuing the invaluable: The economic value of family care giving* (2011 update). Washington, DC: AARP Public Policy Institute. Retrieved from http://assets.aarp.org/rgcenter/ppi/ltc/i51-caregiving.pdf

Han, B., & Haley, W. E. (1999). Family caregiving for patients with stroke. Review and analysis. *Stroke, 30*, 1478–1485.

Houser, A., & Gibson, M. J. (2008). *Valuing the invaluable: The economic value of family care giving* (2008 update). Washington, DC: AARP Public Policy Institute. Retrieved from http://assets.aarp.org/rgcenter/il/i13_caregiving.pdf

Keith, C. (1995). Family care giving systems: Models, resources and values. *Journal of Marriage and the Family, 57*, 179–189.

Kiecott-Glaser, J. K., Preacher, K. J., MacCallum, R. C., Aikinson, C., Malarkey, W. B., & Glaser, R. (2003). Chronic stress and age-related increases in the proinflammatory cytokine IL-6. *Proceedings of the National Academy of Sciences, 100*, 9090–9095. doi:10.1073/pnas,1531903100

Kim, Y., Baker, F., Spillers, R. L., & Wellisch, D. K. (2006). Psychological adjustment of cancer caregivers with multiple roles. *Psycho-oncology, 15*, 795–804.

Kim, Y., & Schulz, R. (2008). Family caregivers' strains: Comparative analysis of cancer caregiver with dementia, diabetes, and frail elderly caregiving. *Journal of Aging and Health, 20*, 483–503.

Kramer, B. J. (2002). Men caregivers: An overview. In B. J. Kramer & E. H. Thompson (Eds.), *Men caregivers: Theory, research, and service implications* (pp. 3–19). New York, NY: Springer.

Kreutzer, J. S., Marwitz, J. H., & Kepler, K. (1992). Traumatic brain injury: Family response and outcome. *Archives of Physical Medicine and Rehabilitation, 73*, 771–778.

Lai, D. W. (2012). Effect of financial costs on caregiving burden of family caregivers of older adults. *Sage Open.* doi:10.1177/2158244012470467

McCann, J. J., Hebert, L. E., Beckett, L. A., Morris, M. C., Scherr, P. A., & Evans, D. A. (2000). Comparison of informal caregiving by black and white older adults in a community population. *Journal of the American Geriatrics Society 48*, 1612–1617.

Metropolitan Life Insurance Company. (1999). *The MetLife Juggling Act Study: Balancing caregiving with work and the costs involved.* Westport, CT: Author.

National Alliance for Caregiving in collaboration with AARP. (2004). *Caregiving in the U.S.* Retrieved from http://www.caregiving.org/data/04finalreport.pdf

National Alliance for Caregiving in collaboration with AARP. (2009). *Caregiving in the U.S.* Retrieved from http://www.caregiving.org/data/Caregiving_in_the_US_2009_full_report.pdf

National Alliance for Caregiving & Evercare. (2006). *Evercare study caregivers in decline: A close-up look at health risks of caring for a loved one.* Retrieved from http://www.caregiving.org/data/Caregivers%20in%20Decline%20StudyFINAL-lowres.pdf

National Alliance for Caregiving & the United Hospital Fund. (2005). *Young caregivers in the U.S.* Retrieved from http://www.caregiving.org/data/youngcaregivers.pdf

Payne, J. C. (1992). Communications and aging: A case for understanding African Americans who are elderly. *ASHA, 34,* 40–44.

Payne, J. C. (2009, March 3). Supporting family caregivers: The role of speech language pathologists and audiologists. *The ASHA Leader.* Retrieved from http://www.asha.org/Publication/leader/2009/090303/090303d.htm

Reinhard, S. C., Feinberg, L., & Choula, R. (2011). *The challenges of family caregiving: What experts say needs to be done.* Washington, DC: AARP Public Policy Institute. Retrieved from http://www.aarp.org/content/dam/aarp/research/public_policy_institute/ltc/012/Spotlight-Paper-Meeting-the-Challenges-of-Family-Caregiving-AARPppi-ltc.pdf

Reinhard, S. C., Given, B., Petlick, N. H., & Bemis, A. (2008). Supporting family caregivers in providing care. In R. G. Hughes (Ed.), *Patient safety and quality: An evidence-based handbook for nurses* (Chapter 14). Rockville, MD: Agency for Healthcare Research and Quality. Retrieved from http://www.ncbi.nlm.nih.gov/books/NBK2665/

Reinhard, S. C., Levine, C., & Samis, S. (2012). *Home alone: Family caregivers providing complex chronic care. AARP with the United Hospital Fund.* Retrieved from http://www.aarp.org/content/dam/aarp/research/public_policy_institue/ltc/012/home-alone-family-caregivers-providing-complex-chroniccare-inbrief-AARP-ppi-health.pdf

Spillers, R. L., Wellisch, D. K., Kim, Y., Matthews, B. A., & Baker, F. (2008). Family caregivers and guilt in the context of cancer care. *Psychosomatics, 49,* 511–519.

Stucki, B. R., & Mulvey, J. (2000). *Can aging baby boomers avoid the nursing home? Long-term care insurance for aging in place* (p. 15). Washington, DC: American Council of Life Insurers. Retrieved from http://www.logos4me.com/Long%20Term%20Care/Can%20BB%20Avoi%20Home.pdf

The Commonwealth Fund. (1999). *Informal caregiving* (Fact Sheet, May). Retrieved from http://www.commonwealthfund.org/~/media/files/publications/databrief/1999/may/informal-caregiving/caregiving_fact_sheet-pdf.pdf

Thompson, H. S., & Ryan, A. (2009). The impact of stroke consequences on spousal relationships from the perspective of the person with stroke. *Journal of Clinical Nursing, 18*, 1803–1811.

U.S. Department of Health and Human Services. (n.d.). *Administration on Aging (AoA) National Family Caregiver Support Program (OAA Title IIIE)*. Retrieved from http://www.aoa.gov/aoa_programs/hcltc/caregiver/index.aspx#10Anni

U.S. Department of Labor. (2014). *Wage and hour division. The Family and Medical Leave Act of 1993, as amended.* Retrieved from http://www.dol.gov/whd/fmla/fmlaAmended.htm

Whitlatch, C. J., Schur, D., Noelker, L. S., Ejaz, F. K., & Looman, W. J. (2001). The stress process of family caregiving in institutional settings. *The Gerontologist, 41*, 462–473.

Wood, R. L., Liossi, C., & Wood, L. (2005). The impact of head injury neurobehavioral sequelae on personal relationships: Preliminary findings. *Brain Injury, 19*, 845–851.

Youngmee, K., Wellisch, D. K., & Spiller, R. L. (2008). Effects of psychological stress on quality of life of adult daughters and their mothers with cancer. *Psycho-oncology, 17*, 1129–1136.

Zarit, S. H., Reever, K. E., & Bach-Peterson, J. (1980). Relatives of the impaired elderly: Correlates of feelings of burden. *The Gerontologist, 20*, 649–655.

3

Diversity Among Caregivers

Joan C. Payne

The preponderance of the literature on family caregivers addresses the needs and concerns of persons in the general population. From the research data, caregiving has many benefits; however, the work of caregiving exacts a heavy toll on all caregivers regardless of their ethnic or cultural identity. While all caregivers are subjected to many of the same stressors, there are differences in how caregivers use formal or informal resources to deliver care, in the belief systems about the obligation for care, and in the perceptions of burdens of caregiving based upon their cultural worldviews.

Cultural and Ethnic Diversity in Caregiving

Cultural and ethnic groups are not homogeneous in language, income, degree of acculturation, education, or adherence to traditions. Just as there are individuals who are living at or below the poverty line, there are those within each ethnic or cultural group who are well educated and financially stable. There are also those who are open to using external resources when needed, have a large family or social support network available to alleviate caregiver strain, or are able to engage in caregiving and attend to their own needs. Despite these intragroup differences, there are some cultural similarities in areas of caregiver stress and coping strategies among caregivers from diverse groups.

Filial obligation (filial piety) and cultural traditions are often the primary reasons that a family member or friend accepts caregiver responsibilities. Within some communities, the prevalence of caregiving is higher than in others. It is estimated that 21% of the U.S. population age 18 and older provides unpaid care to friends or relatives 18 and older. This translates into 44,443,800 caregivers in the United States. While the prevalence of caregiving among non-Hispanic whites and African Americans is 21%, it is slightly lower among Asian American and Hispanic populations (18% and 16%, respectively) (National Alliance for Caregiving in collaboration with AARP, 2009).

Cultural history and traditions influence caregiver perception about the quality of life during caregiving. Cultural variations in the caregiving experience associated with membership in a particular racial or ethnic group were the major areas of discussions among focus group participants interviewed by Scharlach and her associates (2006). Three primary themes emerged which explain, in part, how cultural groups may differ. These are reported by caregivers to be the following:

- Group experiences of adversity and discrimination which affect the caregiving experience
- Caregiving behaviors and norms that differentiate one's own group from the majority culture
- Change in natural support networks because of transitions from cultural norms in one country to more acculturated views of other generations over time

Issues of familism, mistrust of the formal sources of support for caregivers, and service barriers such as language differences and perceptions that formal sources are often culturally inappropriate were also shared during the discussion groups.

The following describes some of the documented differences between caregivers from diverse cultural and ethnic groups. In this section, the role of tradition and cultural expectation are highlighted to explain patterns of coping with caregiver stressors.

Major Differences Between Non-Hispanic White Caregivers and Other Ethnic Groups

Cultural expectations help to define caregiving roles more concisely, but they can also produce depression, guilt, and anger. A review of the literature on diversity in caregiving suggests that cultural expectations of care, such as filial obligation, may lessen stress but may determine how much burden the caregiver feels. Tradition and cultural expectations, therefore, may cause an individual to feel that there was no choice in accepting the role of a caregiver. Although familism is culturally and socially popular, traditional beliefs in the caregiving role can lead to negative psychological consequences for a caregiver.

Perhaps for these reasons, religious organizations and the tribe are tremendous sources of support and comfort during caregiving (Scharlach et al., 2006). The perceptions of burden of care manifest as reports of poorer physical health and depression. For example, African American caregiving women report experiencing less stress, burden, and depression than non-Hispanic white caregivers because of cultural expectations, but they report worse physical health (Cuellar, 2002; Haley et al., 2004). Hispanic and Asian American caregivers may accept caregiving responsibilities because of filial obligation and cultural expectations but exhibit more depression than non-Hispanic white caregivers (Haley et al., 2004).

As a group, ethnic minority caregivers provide more care than their non-Hispanic white counterparts (Hughes, Tyler, Danner, & Carter, 2009). Pinquart and Sörensen (2005) report additional differences among ethnic caregivers based upon a meta-analysis of 116 empirical studies:

- Ethnic minority caregivers made less use of professional support services than did non-Hispanic white caregivers.
- Ethnic minority caregivers have a lower socioeconomic status, are more likely to receive support from family members and friends, provide more

care than non-Hispanic white caregivers, and have stronger filial obligation beliefs than non-Hispanic white caregivers.

- All ethnic minority caregiving groups report worse physical health than the non-Hispanic white caregivers report experiencing.

The main reason for all of these divergences, research suggests, is that cultural perspectives differ across ethnic groups and may impact caregiver experiences in several domains, including perceptions of the caregiving role, use of support services, acculturation, and clinical presentations and interactions. In addition, psychological characteristics often predict adjustment among family members in a theoretically consistent and interpretable manner (Valle, Yamada, & Barrio, 2004).

Others (Mahoney, Cloutterbuck, Neary, & Zhan, 2005) have reported several interesting cultural differences between African Americans, Latinos, and Chinese American caregivers of persons with Alzheimer's dementia. Specifically, African Americans turn to their ministers for information, Latinos turn to their friends, whereas Chinese Americans seek information from regional health centers. As the disease progresses, each ethnic group uses a different strategy to cope with the changes brought on by the disease.

Ethnic differences are also found with regard to the care recipient. Among people aged 70 and older who require care, non-Hispanic whites are the most likely to receive help from their spouses; Hispanics are the most likely to receive help from their adult children; and African Americans are the most likely to receive help from a nonfamily member (National Academy on an Aging Society, 2000). The following discussion speaks to some additional cultural differences in caregiving which have been observed by researchers.

Ethnic Group Identification and Caregiving

Non-Hispanic Whites

Although the terms *white, Caucasian*, and *Anglo Americans* are used interchangeably in the literature, the term *non-Hispanic whites* here refers to those to have their roots in Western, Southern, and Eastern Europe. The National Alliance for Caregiving in collaboration with AARP (2009) reports that 26,177,500 persons of European descent are caring for others over age 50 in this country (2009) from a national total of 32,337,000 caregivers.

Older non-Hispanic whites are more likely to live with and care for a spouse; however, there are strong kinship ties within families and many will depend on adult children in times of illness to provide instrumental support. As a group, non-Hispanic whites tend to have the highest income, report being more comfortable with using outside health care services, including support groups, than their nonwhite age cohorts and have the highest percentage of regular home health care (Karlin, Weil, & Gould, 2012). They are least likely to underuse health services as part of their caregiving because of cost or lack of insurance (National Academy on an Aging Society, 2000). The same is less true for African American and Hispanic caregivers who report more caregiving responsibilities and less reliance on institutional care and other outside services.

An earlier study (Gelfand, 1981) describes intragroup differences among non-Hispanic whites as a function of cultural uniqueness in the nature of the local community, religion, or national origin. Gelfand (1981) described sharing intimate concerns with family members as more characteristic of the white ethnics (e.g., Jews, Italians, and Slavs). Friends and relatives play a more important role in obtaining resource support for Italian and Polish American women. Italian older adults are more likely to continue to live in ethnic communities, compared to Irish or Polish Americans. Church- or temple-sponsored services are used more by elderly Greeks, Italians, and Jews. Jewish older adults are more comfortable with formal support services, like Meals on Wheels, than any other groups. Later research using focus groups (Scharlach et al., 2006) found that Russian caregivers report that their care recipients were comfortable attending an adult day health care (ADHC) or a regional center program for persons with developmental disabilities.

Caregivers' roles in caring for others are discussed in Chapter 2. Differences are noted between non-Hispanic white caregivers and their nonwhite ethnic cohorts in the areas of age, educational achievement, socioeconomic status, and perception of caregiver burden. Non-Hispanic white caregivers are more likely to be over age 65, have a college degree and some graduate education, earn more money, and report that their level of burden in caregiving is minimal when compared to African American and Hispanic caregivers. It is thought that greater longevity of care recipients contributes to the older age of non-Hispanic white caregivers. In summary, non-Hispanic white caregivers:

- are older than other caregivers and care for older adults;
- are generally comfortable seeking and using outside help;
- have a larger income than that of ethnic caregivers;
- are affected by the burden of care but not to the degree as ethnic caregivers are affected;
- are more likely to be educated;
- are likely to depend on adult children for instrumental support;
- are more likely to be married, living with a spouse;
- are more likely to care for a spouse; and
- are more often women.

African American Caregivers

African American elder adults continue to live in the community, with and because of the support and assistance of their family members. Presently, there are 3,657,100 African American caregivers in the United States caring for an adult over age 50 out of a total of 5,119,400 estimated caregivers (National Alliance for Caregiving in collaboration with AARP, 2009). By the year 2030, there may be as many as 7.3 million African American elders in the United States, signaling an increased need for African American caregivers.

African American caregivers are an average of 45 years old and more likely to be single, never married (28% versus 15% of caregivers overall or 12% of non-Hispanic white caregivers) women. These caregivers are more likely to provide assistance with three or more ADLs. Many have an annual income of less than $50,000 and are more likely to be low-income than non-

Hispanic white caregivers (National Alliance for Caregiving & Evercare, 2006).

Care recipients frequently live with the care provider, are usually over age 75 (64%), and are more likely to have long-term illnesses such as dementia (28%) and stroke (12% compared to 7% for other groups). While African American caregivers provide many of the same activities as their counterparts in other groups (instrumental activities of daily living [IADLs], transportation, finances, domestic chores), they are more likely to give medications (51% for African Americans as compared with 35% for non-Hispanic whites) and spend on average 20.6 hours per week in this role. In addition, 66% of African American caregivers are employed full or part time (National Alliance for Caregiving & Evercare, 2006).

African American families adhere closely to values of responsibility to family, the extended family network, and home care for relatives for as long as feasible. As a result, African Americans traditionally maintain their family members at home rather than place them in nursing home care and have a low use of formal caregiver services. In a cross-sectional study of 521 Midwestern African American women caregivers, Rozario and DeRienzis (2008) found that wife caregivers, caregivers with lower levels of education, and caregivers with lower levels of educational achievement held significantly more traditional caregiving beliefs. These beliefs may help to define who will serve as caregivers but can also place a heavy responsibility on a caregiver who may feel that he or she had few choices. For example, although African American caregivers report lower levels of burden, they have demonstrated higher levels of depression and anxiety when compared to non-Hispanic white caregivers.

African American caregivers also tend to use emotion-focused coping which increases emotional distress. These caregivers report that they frequently use prayer to cope. However, having poor caregiving relationships, being younger, being unemployed or underemployed, and having lower levels of education can affect self-rated health and mastery. Perceptions of poor health and feelings of not being in control have been associated with increased burden, higher levels of depression, and perceived stress in caregivers. This may explain, in part, why African American families delay confirming a diagnosis of Alzheimer's disease in a loved one until the disease is well advanced (Hughes, Tyler, Danner, & Carter, 2009).

Churches in African American communities have long been recognized as sources of instrumental and emotional support. Comparative studies of cultural/ethnic contexts of families who are caregiving often cite religion as a salient factor in family adjustment. In particular, caregivers of adults with chronic/disabling illnesses report that church support is critical for coping with the stressors of caregiving. Pickett-Schenk (2002) examined the effectiveness of church-based support groups and found that respondents' improved knowledge and morale outcomes suggest that church-based support groups may be a valuable coping resource for African American families of disabled adults. In summary, African American caregivers are seen to be

- reluctant to place loved ones in institutional care or to use formal supports,
- more often women,
- reliant on an emotional coping style and prayer,
- heavily reliant on friends and church members for support,
- younger than non-Hispanic white caregivers and often with limited resources,
- less reliant on outside or agency support,
- more comfortable with church-sponsored resources, and
- invested in traditional norms for caregiving.

Hispanic Caregivers

There are an estimated 8,147,000 Hispanic caregivers in the United States (National Alliance for Caregiving & Evercare, 2006), 2,800,700 of whom are caring for an adult over age 50. Hispanics are projected to have the longest life expectancy of any ethnic group. Hispanic caregivers are an average age of 43 years old and are significantly younger than non-Hispanic white and African American caregivers. They are also less likely to be married than non-Hispanic white caregivers, and many report that they have an annual income of less than $50,000. Hispanic caregivers are more likely to report that there are children or grandchildren living in their households who are age 18 and under. Just under three quarters (74%) of Hispanic caregivers are female, caring for a loved one whose average age is 62. Most of the care recipients are female (American Psychological Association, 2008).

A significant number of the 1,007 Hispanic caregivers interviewed for a 2008 study of Hispanic caregivers reported that their family or ancestors originated in Mexico (75%). Others come from Central America (5%), Spain (4%), South America (3%), Puerto Rico (2%), Cuba (2%), or the Dominican Republic (2%). While one in three of the Hispanic caregivers has lived his or her entire life in the United States (36%), four in ten have lived less than half of their life in the United States (39%) (National Alliance for Caregiving & Evercare, 2006).

Hispanic cultures and kinship patterns provide strong support for needy elders (Cuellar, 1990). Hispanic elderly are likely to live within the context of large, extended families, or live in close proximity (Becerra & Shaw, 1984). Hispanic families exchange emotional, financial, and social support, as well as assistance in the routine tasks of daily living during illness. Even in situations where extended family members are in separate households, grandparents, uncles and aunts, siblings, cousins, in-laws, and godparents often provide nurture, guidance, and support (Ho, 1987). Like African Americans, the church is an important source of comfort and support for Hispanic caregivers (Karlin et al., 2012; Krause & Bastida, 2011).

Diabetes is the major reason why Hispanic caregivers say their recipients need care, and it is almost twice as prevalent a reason for them as it is for non-Hispanics (15% versus 8%). Cancer, old age, and arthritis are the next most common (7% each). Although Alzheimer's or mental confusion is cited by only 6% of Hispanic caregivers as the primary reason why their care recipients need care, a total of 23% say their loved ones suffer from this condition. Hispanics are reluctant to place their care recipients in institutional care, preferring to care for them in their homes (American Psychological Association, 2008).

Several researchers (Valle, Yamada, & Barrio, 2004; Villa, Cuellar, Gamel, & Yeo, 1993) have noted that Cuban, Spanish, and Puerto Rican caregivers are often female daughters, daughters-in-law, or female non-kin. In most cases, however, the entire family will be closely involved in the health care decisions that affect older persons.

Hispanic family caregivers tend to be in more intensive caregiving situations with 63% in high burden situations compared to 51% of non-Hispanic caregivers. Also, Hispanic caregivers spend more hours per week giving care (on average 37 hours versus 31 hours) and provide a greater number of activities of daily living known as personal care (2.6 versus 1.9) than non-Hispanic white caregivers. A higher percentage of Hispanic caregivers live with their loved one (43%) as compared to 32% of non-Hispanic caregivers (American Psychological Association, 2008). In summary, Hispanic caregivers are seen to be

- younger in age than other caregivers and often with limited resources,
- likely to have children and/or grandchildren in their households,
- diverse in country of origin,
- reluctant to place care recipients in institutional care,
- more often women,
- more likely to have extended family support,
- inclusive about family opinion in health care decisions,
- reliant upon traditional caregiving roles and the church, and
- bearers of heavy responsibility for care.

Asian American Caregivers

Currently, it is estimated that there are 1,527,500 Asian American caregivers in the United States, 1,273,900 of whom are caring for persons over age 50 (National Alliance for Caregiving in collaboration with AARP, 2009). Asian American caregivers are both men (48%) and women (52%). This is a significant difference from the national average where 72.5% of informal caregivers are women. Like Hispanic caregivers, Asian Americans are extremely diverse in national origin, language, and culture from East and Southeast Asia, the Indian subcontinent, Polynesia, Melanesia, and Micronesia.

The national average age of caregivers is 46; however, Asian American caregivers tend to be younger (mean age of 39.1

years). Approximately 62% of the Asian caregivers interviewed had postsecondary school education; 77% were employed full or part time (versus 65% for other groups); and 61% have a household income of more than $30,000 (median household income $45,000 versus $35,000) (National Alliance for Caregiving in collaboration with AARP, 2009).

Asian Americans spend an average of 15.1 hours per week providing care compared to other groups who spend over 18 hours. Asian American caregivers tend to live in the same home with the care recipients (35% versus 19% of non-Hispanic white caregivers), and 51.1% have one or more children under age 18 living in the household. This may explain why 61% of caregivers feel that other family members, especially daughters-in-law (11%), are sharing in the caring process and why they feel caregiving does not compromise their family relationships (American Psychological Association, 2008).

Filial piety mandates that sons and daughters of older, frail parents are obligated to provide care (Lai, 2010). Although filial piety is seen in other groups, among some Asian American groups, this construct is not gender specific. This is a major difference in gender roles in caregiving from other ethnic groups. To summarize, Asian Americans caregivers as a group are

- diverse in country of origin and languages,
- more likely to have a college education,
- more likely to have an income comparable to non-Hispanic whites,
- hold that filial piety applies to both males and females,
- are younger than the national average for caregivers,
- provide at least 15.1 hours a week in care, and
- are likely to be comfortable with seeking outside support.

American Indian/Alaska Native (AI/AN) Caregivers

There are 2.1 million American Indians and Alaskan Natives in the United States today, and that number is projected to double by the year 2050. There are 545 federally recognized tribes and 100 more that do not have federal recognition. The rural native population has a higher concentration of children and elders than does the urban population. Many in the 18-to-55 age group migrate to cities or other areas in search of employment only to return when they become elders (Goins et al., 2011).

Most American Indian families apply an age-old practice in which certain individuals (family members or chosen individuals) are given or assume a duty to care for an elder or disabled individual—the word "caregiver" is simply not commonly used. Caregiver connotes a "job" instead of a customary duty or responsibility (Goins et al., 2011).

There are few studies on caregivers within tribal nations. It is estimated that the average age of an AI/AN caregiver is between 45 and 54 years of age. Looking only at North Dakota Indians, the typical caregiver is female, and taking care of a spouse or mother over the age of 60 who has physical disabilities or cognitive impairment (National Resource Center on Native American Aging, 2004). About 16.4% of the general U.S. population is caring for an older adult, compared to 17.6% of the AI/AN population (McGuire, Okoro, Goins, & Anderson, 2008). Like many people of other racial/ethnic groups, AI/AN families want to care for their elders and the elders want to remain in their homes and have family care for them as long as possible (Okoro et al., 2007).

Many current or prospective American Indian caregivers tend to be younger than the general population. In one study (Hennessy & John, 1996), the average age of the caregiver was 50. They performed at least 4 hours a day of direct care, or 50%. Most were daughters caring for parents and most worked at least half time. Many caregivers served disabled elders while they were still raising children and grandchildren. In another study, 60% had provided care for 6 months to 3 years, 17% between 3 and 5 years, and 20% for over five years. The majority of these individuals balance dual care responsibilities for an elder and a child or grandchild and are less likely to be married or providing spousal care when compared with the general population (Center for Rural Health, 2003).

A recent cross-sectional investigation of 5,207 American Indian adults residing on two closely related Lakota Sioux reservations in the Northern Plains and one American Indian community in the Southwest examined the relationship between culture and traditional healing practices (Goins et al., 2011). Of those sampled, 17% reported being caregivers. In both the Northern Plains and Southwest, caregiving was positively correlated with younger age, being a woman, having a larger household size, attending and participating in Native events, and knowledge about and endorsement of traditional healing practices. In both regions, attendance and participation in Native events and engagement in traditional healing practices were associated with increased odds of caregiving because greater cultural identity and engagement in traditional healing practices were related to more effective care. Speaking some Native language increased the odds of an individual being delegated as a caregiver in the Northern Plains.

One concern for the AI/AN population is that there is an out-migration from the reservations to urban areas for jobs leaving a potentially smaller pool of prospective caregivers. Garrett and colleagues (Garrett, Baldridge, Benson, & McGuire, 2008; Garrett & McGuire, 2008) developed the Caregiver Ratio Index (CRI), which is an algorithm that defines how many potential caregivers exist for every frail elder by tribe. The higher the CRI, the higher the number of potential caregivers there are for each frail elder. Lower CRI ratings were aligned with those Native communities that showed migration to the South, reflecting national trends and probably motivated by the search for employment.

For the American Indian/Alaskan Native (AI/AN) population, taking care of an elder is a continuation of an ancient custom of extended family and lifelong care for family. Indian family caregivers are similar to non-Indian caregivers in many ways; however, the resources available to them are much more limited than for non-Indian caregivers. In addition, eligibility criteria for long-term care services are often couched in language that is not culturally sensitive. American Indian/Alaska Native caregivers are likely to be

- reliant on cultural identity as a means to identify caregivers;
- mostly women, with limited resources;
- younger than non-Hispanic white caregivers;
- assigned their caregiving role because of tribal traditions;
- comfortable with traditional health practices; and
- less likely to seek resources outside of the tribe.

Middle Eastern Americans

There is little information available about Middle Eastern Americans and caregiving. What exists are limited descriptions about Muslim doctrine, family structure, and health care (Galanti, 2008; Sinunu, Yount, & El Afify, 2009). Caregiving roles, stressors, and responsibilities can be implied from what is written about the cultures of some countries in the Middle East. Although the general term *Middle Eastern* is used in this country to mean all peoples who live in Middle Eastern countries, persons from some countries share more cultural commonalities than others, for example, Arab, Egyptian, and Iranian Americans. Not all persons from the Middle East are Muslims; however, the vast majority of persons are. The American view of individual responsibility and control over life's events is in direct opposition to the Middle Eastern view of responsibility for health and well-being. According to the Middle Eastern perspective, the family is the context through which health care is delivered. Family members indulge the patient and assume responsibility for all decisions. The Koran puts forth gender-specific role responsibilities for family members (Salimbene, 2000).

Middle Eastern Americans as a group have great respect for Western medicine and are likely to accept the advice of physicians without question. However, unlike the American practice of full disclosure of diagnosis and possible complications, Middle Eastern physicians will most likely withhold information about a grave diagnosis or the full details of a surgical procedure. Similarly, preoperative instructions are often withheld in the belief that they will cause needless anxiety. Patients are not usually interested in participating in medical decision making. Medical successes are attributed to the expertise of the physician, while failures are attributed to the will of Allah (Galanti, 2008).

Women are most often the primary caregivers. The immediate and extended family forms the most important social institution in the Middle East. Parents are expected to care for children until they are married, and children are not only expected to remain in close contact with parents after marriage but also to care for aged parents as long as they live; however, these relationships are likely undergoing change in Egypt because of modernization (Yount & Khadr, 2008). The implications for

Egyptian American families are unclear. However, Soliman and Almotgly (2011) found that Egyptian families who care for persons with HIV/AIDS are both stigmatized and heavily burdened with few resources.

In the traditional Iranian family, households are often multigenerational. As a result, nursing home placement for a loved one is perceived as unacceptable and a failure of filial piety. Older Iranians in need of care, therefore, are more likely to be cared for by a loved one in their family (Deljavan, 2013). In many Middle Eastern families, the family structure is patriarchal in form and even adult children are expected to submit to the father's authority.

According to Khalaila and Litwin (2011), the vast majority of Arab American family caregivers indicate that they would like to be cared for by family members. However, location, particularly for those living in urban areas, is negatively correlated with preference for family care but positively correlated with preferences for more formal care. However, these associations are mediated by the extent of filial piety and caregiving burden. Those who expressed the highest levels of filial piety are most likely to prefer family care in the future as contrasted with help from formal supports. Perceptions of caregiving burden greatly influence preferences for future formal care.

Iranian American caregivers have identified formal service barriers, such as language or cultural or religious appropriateness, as consistent impediments to access to caregiver support services. Additionally, an overriding sense of duty and responsibility in caregiving is also a barrier because it causes caregivers to become reluctant to seek assistance. Thus, Iranian caregivers are less likely to utilize services that might otherwise ease the burden of caregiving (Azar & Dadvar, 2007). In conclusion, Middle Eastern American caregivers are likely to

- be strong proponents of within-family caregiving,
- be women,
- be less accepting of external caregiver support services,
- view nursing home placement as unacceptable,
- be respectful of Western medicine,
- prefer not to have full disclosure of illness diagnoses, and
- be indulgent of the care recipient.

Discussion of Differences

Table 3–1 illustrates some of the major factors that can differentiate caregivers across ethnic and cultural groups. As can be seen,
women provide the majority of care for care recipients, with the
exception of Asian Americans/Pacific Islanders for whom filial
piety is not gender specific. It is apparent that poor women
have the greatest burden in caregiving. Non-Hispanic whites and
some Asian Americans are more likely to have adequate financial
resources and have a greater level of comfort with accessing
resources outside of the family network. However, African and
Hispanic Americans are more likely to have a more extensive
support system of friends, church members, and family to assist
them in caregiving, but often do not use or have the financial
means to use outside resources frequently to assist in the responsibilities of caregiving. African, Hispanic, and Middle Eastern
Americans may be more comfortable with accessing community
and religious-based resources.

At the conclusion of this chapter, resources that are appropriate for all ethnic groups are included as are websites identified as specific for diverse ethnic groups. Clinicians may use this
information to inform their patients with communication and
swallowing issues about culturally appropriate resources that
are available.

Summary

Just as there is diversity within the society, there is diversity in
caregiving roles, cultural identification with caregiving responsibilities, caregiver age, care recipient age, available resources,
and caregiver needs. Acceptance of traditional roles of caregiving
has the positive effect of ensuring that disabled adults will have
support from persons within their family constellation, whether
kin, extended family, or friends. On the negative side, however, heavy caregiving responsibilities, limited financial means,
advanced age of the care recipient, and few resources to sustain
caregivers or provide them relief can have a deleterious effect
on the health and well-being of the caregiver and, ultimately,

Table 3–1. Summary of Group Characteristics of Caregivers by Ethnicity

Ethnic Group	Primarily Women	Women or Men (Filial Piety)	Comfortable With External Supports	Adequacy of Income	Extended Support Network	High Level of Burden
Non-Hispanic Whites	X		X	X	X	
African Americans	X				X	X
Hispanic Americans	X				X	X
Native Americans/Alaska Natives	X				X	X
Asian Americans/Pacific Islanders	X	X	X	X	X	X
Middle Eastern Americans	X			X	X	X

the care recipient. To assist clinicians in identifying resources for ethnic caregivers, a list of resources applicable to the general population and sorted by ethnic group is found at the end of this chapter.

Differences in use of formal caregiver resources can be seen between non-Hispanic white caregivers and those from other ethnic backgrounds. Whether these differences are attributable to level of comfort, knowledge about resources, perceptions of cultural appropriateness, or differing views on health care and disease stigma, it is clear that those caregivers who are unable to ease their responsibilities with outside support are the most vulnerable to physical and emotional stressors that can impair their own health and well-being.

A limitation in interpreting research data is that diverse caregivers who provide responses in focus groups or in surveys are generally already using support, community, or health-related resources. The results may not be generalizable to a larger population. The richness of subject sampling may be compromised because of the number of undocumented persons who may refuse to be interviewed or who are eliminated from data analyses. Nonetheless, the available data suggest trends in differences between and even within ethnic and cultural groups. Specifically, a major trend is that caregivers with fewer financial resources and limited access to external resources reported a higher level of perceived burden in caregiving. It is these most vulnerable caregivers to whom speech-language pathologists and audiologists should pay particular attention.

Caregiver Resources for All Ethnic Groups

National Family Caregivers Association
The National Family Caregivers Association, a caregiver membership organization, provides services in the areas of information and education, support and validation, public awareness, and advocacy for caregivers.

> http://www.nfcacares.org
> 10605 Concord St., Suite 501

Kensington, MD 20895-2504
(800) 896-3650
info@nfcacares.org

National Alliance for Caregiving
The National Alliance for Caregiving, a partnership of several aging organizations, conducts research, develops national projects, and works to increase public awareness of the issues of family caregiving for older Americans.

http://www.caregiving.org
4720 Montgomery Lane, Suite 642
Bethesda, MD 20814
(301) 718-8444

National Hotline for Physician Reporting of Elder Abuse and Neglect

(800) 490-8505

The Eldercare Locator
The Locator provides information about community assistance for seniors in communities across the United States. The toll-free number is a public service sponsored by the U.S. Administration on Aging.

http://www.eldercare.gov
(800) 677-1116

The National Aging Information Center
An informative brochure describing the Eldercare Locator service is available free through the National Aging Information Center.

330 Independence Avenue, S.W.
Washington, DC 20201
(202) 619-7501

U.S. Administration on Aging
The Administration on Aging (AoA) is the focal point for services to seniors in the U.S. Department of Health and Human Services. Through a nationwide network of state and area agencies on aging and tribal organizations, AoA plans, develops, and supports

comprehensive in-home and community services including information and referral services, job and volunteer opportunities, senior center and day care center programs, transportation, a nationwide congregate and home-delivered meals program, and homemaker and home health aide services in addition to legal services, nursing home ombudsmen services, and counseling programs to assist seniors if they are abused, neglected, or exploited.

> http://www.aoa.gov
> 330 Independence Avenue, SW
> Washington, DC 20201
> (202) 619-0724

Office of Disability, Aging, and Long-Term Care Policy, ASPE, HHS

The Office of Disability, Aging, and Long-Term Care Policy (DALTCP), under the Assistant Secretary for Planning and Evaluation (ASPE), conducts policy research on informal caregiving for the U.S. Department of Health and Human Services (HHS). For a list of recent research publications on informal caregiving, contact DALTCP.

> http://www.aspe.hhs.gov
> DALTCP/ASPE/DHHS
> Room 424E, H.H. Humphrey Building
> 200 Independence Avenue, SW
> Washington, DC 20201
> (202) 690-6443
> daltcp2@oaspe.dhhs.gov

The Resource Directory for Older People

The Resource Directory for Older People is available on the AoA website (http://www.aoa.dhhs.gov) and is also available in hard copy. It is intended to serve a wide audience including older people and their families, health and legal professionals, social service providers, librarians, researchers, and others with an interest in the field of aging. The directory contains contact information for organizations that provide information and other resources on matters relevant to the needs of older persons. The directory is a joint project of the Administration on Aging and the National Institute on Aging. A hard copy of the directory is available for $11.00 from:

> Superintendent of Documents
> P.O. Box 371954
> Pittsburgh, PA 15250-7954
> Publication Number - 0106200145-6
> (202) 512-1800

Rosalynn Carter Institute for Caregiving

Provides caregiver support to individuals through education and advocacy through local, state, and national partnerships.

> http://www.rosalynncarter.org
> 800 GSW Drive
> Georgia Southwestern State University
> Americus, GA 31709-4379
> Phone: (229) 928-1234
> Fax: (229) 931-2663

Caregiver Resources Specific to Ethnic Groups

African Americans

The Internet Stroke Center: Caregiving Guide for African Americans

> http://www.strokecenter.org/patients/
> caregiver-and-patient-resources/
> caregiving-guide-for-african-americans/introduction/

Ethnic Elders Care: African Americans and Dementia

> http://www.ethnicelderscare.net
> (925) 372-2105

Alzheimer's Association

Annual African American Caregivers Forum

> http://www.alz.org/alzwa/in_my_community_13864.asp
> 24/7 Helpline: (800) 272-3900

American Indians/Alaska Natives

National Resource Center for American Indian, Alaska Native, and Native Hawaiian Elders

http://www.elders.uaa.alaska.edu/about.htm
(907) 786-4440

Administration on Aging: Native American Programs

http://www.olderindians.aoa.gov/announcements.cfm
One Massachusetts Avenue
Washington, DC 20201
(202) 401-4634

Alu Like, Inc.
Native American Caregivers Support Program

http://www.alulike.org/services/kumu_native.html
(808) 535-6700

U.S. Department of Health & Human Services
Native American Caregiver Support Services

http://www.hhs.gov/grantsforecast/cfda/health/
planning/aoa16.html
(877) 696-6775

The Otoe Missouria Tribe
Native American Family Caregiver Support Program

http://www.omtribe.org/index.php?
elder-care-caregiver-support-services
Leda Green, Caregiver
(580) 723-4466

Hispanic Americans

Alzheimer's Association in Spanish

http://www.alz.org/hispanic/overview-sp.asp
(800) 272-3900

Healthfinder Español
Resource for finding the best government and nonprofit health and human services information.

> http://www.healthfinder.gov/espanol/
> 1101 Wootton Parkway
> Rockville, MD 20852
> healthfinder@hhs.gov

Hispanics and Dementia

> Department of Psychiatry, University of California
> http://www.ethnicelderscare.net/
> ethnicity&dementiahis.htm
> Rita Hargrave
> (925) 372-2105

La Raza

> Janet Murguía, President and CEO
> Raul Yzaguirre Building
> http://www.nclr.org
> 1126 16th Street, NW, Suite 600
> Washington, DC 20036-4845
> (202) 785-1670

National Alliance for Hispanic Health

> http://www.hispanichealth.org
> Jane Delgado
> (202) 387-5000

Older Adult Family Center

> Stanford School of Medicine
> http://www.med.standford.edu/oac/
> (800) 943-4333

Su Familia: The National Hispanic Family Health Helpline in Spanish

> http://www.hispanichealth.org/helplines.lasso
> (866) 783-2645

Asian Americans/Pacific Islanders

Chinese and Dementia

Department of Psychiatry, University of California
http://www.ethnicelderscare.net/
ethnicity%26dementiachinese.htm
(925) 372-2105

Chinese Community Health Resource Center

http://www.cchrchealth.org
(415) 677-2473

Japanese Americans and Dementia

Department of Psychiatry, University of California
http://www.ethnicelderscare.net/
ethnicity&dementiaasia.htm
(925) 372-2105

Middle Eastern Americans

Islamic Social Services Association

http://www.issausa.org

Association of Muslim Health Professionals

http://www.amhp.us

MCC—Muslim Community Center for Human Services

http://www.mcc-hs.org
(817) 589-9165

Islamic Society of North America

http://www.isna.net

Mosque Cares

http://www.themosquecares.com

Muslim American Society

http://www.masnet.org

Muslim Alliance of North America

http://www.mana-net.org

References

Alzheimer's Association. (n.d.). *Serving Hispanic families: Home and community based services for people with dementia and their caregivers.* Retrieved from http://www.aoa.gov/AoARoot/AoA_Programs/HPW/Alz_Grants/docs/Toolit6_HispanicFamilies.pdf

American Psychological Association. (2008). *Cultural diversity and caregiving.* Retrieved from http://www.apa.org/pi/about/publications/caregivers/faq/cultural-diversity

Azar, A., & Dadvar, S. (2007). Psychoeducational program for Iranian family caregivers living in Northern California. *Clinical Gerontologist, 31,* 95–100.

Becerra, R. L., & Shaw, D. (1984). *The Hispanic elderly: A research reference guide.* New York, NY: Academic Press.

Center for Rural Health. (2003). *National family caregivers support program: North Dakota's support program in North Dakota.* Retrieved from http://www.nrcnaa.org/pdf/CaregiverSupportProgram.pdf

Cuellar, J. B. (1990). *Hispanic American aging: Geriatric education curriculum development for selected health professionals.* Health Resources and Services Administration, Department of Health and Human Services (DHHS Publication No. HRS IP-DV-90-41) (pp. 121–128). Washington, DC: U.S. Government Printing Office.

Cuellar, N. G. (2002). Comparison of African American and Caucasian American female caregivers of rural, post-stroke, bedbound older adults. *Journal of Gerontological Nursing, 28,* 36–45.

Deljavan, S. (2013). *Exploring the Iranian-Canadian family experience of dementia caregiving: A phenomenological study* (Unpublished thesis). University of Western Ontario, Canada.

Galanti, G. A. (2008). *Caring for patients from different cultures* (4th ed., pp. 241–250). Philadelphia, PA: University of Pennsylvania Press.

Garrett, M. D., Baldridge, D., Benson, W. F., & McGuire, L. C. (2008). Missing cohorts of caregivers among American Indian and Alaska native communities. *The HIS Primary Care Provider, 33,* 105–111.

Retrieved from http://www.ihs.gov/publicInfo/publications/Health Provider/issues/PROV0408.pdf

Garrett, M. D., & McGuire, L. C. (2008). Family caregivers declining for American Indians, Alaska Natives. *Aging Today, 11,* 29. Retrieved from http://www.asaging.org/at/at-296/toc.cfm

Gelfand, D. E. (1981). Ethnicity and aging. *Annual Review of Gerontology and Geriatrics, 2,* 91–115.

Goins, R. T., Spencer, S. M., McGuire, L. C., Goldberg, J., Wen, Y., & Henderson, J. A. (2011). Adult caregiving among American Indians: The role of cultural factors. *Gerontologist, 51,* 310–320. doi:10.1093/geront/gnq101

Haley, W. E., Gitlin, L. N., Wisniewski, S. R., Mahoney, D. F., Cood, D. W., Winter, L., . . . Ory, M. (2004). Well-being, appraisal, and coping in African-American and Caucasian dementia caregivers: Findings from the REACH study. *Aging and Mental Health, 8,* 316–329.

Hennessey, C. H., & John, R. J. (1996). American Indian family caregivers' perceptions of burden and needed support services. *Journal of Applied Gerontology, 15,* 275–288.

Ho, M. K. (1987). *Family therapy with ethnic minorities.* Newbury Park, CA: Sage.

Hughes, T., Tyler, K., Danner, D., & Carter, A. (2009). African American caregivers: An exploration of pathways and barriers to a diagnosis of Alzheimer's disease for a family member with dementia. *International Journal of Social Research and Practice, 8,* 95–116.

Karlin, N. J., Weil, J., & Gould, J. (2012). *Comparisons between Hispanic and non-Hispanic white informal caregivers.* Retrieved from http://sgo.sagepub.com/content/2/4/2158244012470108

Khalaila, R., & Litwin, H. (2011). Modernization and future care preferences: A cross-sectional survey of Arab Israeli caregivers. *Journal of Advanced Nursing, 67,* 1614–1624.

Krause, N., & Bastida, E. (2011). Religion, suffering, and self-rated health among older Mexican Americans. *Journals of Gerontology: Social Sciences, 66B,* 207–216.

Lai, D. W. (2010). Filial piety, caregiving appraisal, and caregiving burden. *Research on Aging, 32,* 200–223.

Mahoney, D. F., Cloutterbuck, J., Neary, S., & Zhan, L. (2005). African American, Chinese, and Latino family caregiving impressions of the onset and diagnosis of dementia: Cross-cultural similarities and differences. *Gerontologist, 45,* 783–792.

McGuire, L. C., Okoro, C. A., Goins, R.T., & Anderson, L. A. (2008). Characteristics of American Indian and Alaska Native adult caregivers, behavioral risk factor surveillance system, 2000. *Ethnicity & Disease, 18,* 477–482.

National Academy on an Aging Society. (2000). *Caregiving: Helping the elderly with activity limitations.* Retrieved from https://georgetown .app.box.com/s/1wfvnbl8gwodo6ezf9cb

National Alliance for Caregiving & Evercare. (2006). *Evercare study of caregivers in decline: A close-up look at health risks of caring for a loved one.* Retrieved from http://www.caregiving.org/data/Caregivers %20in%20Decline%20StudyFINAL-lowres.pdf

National Alliance for Caregiving in collaboration with AARP. (2009). *Caregiving in the United States.* Retrieved from http://www.caregiving .org/data/Caregiving_in_the_US_2009_full_report.pdf

National Resource Center on Native American Aging. (2004). *Health literacy review.* Retrieved from http://ruralhealth.und.edu/projects/ nrcnaa/pdf/health_literacy.pdf

Okoro, C. A., Denny, C. H., McGuire, L. C., Balluz, L. S., Goins, R. T., & Mokdad, A. H. (2007). Disability among older American Indians and Alaska Natives: Disparities in prevalence, health-risk behaviors, obesity, and chronic conditions. *Ethnicity & Disease, 17,* 686–692.

Pickett-Schenk, S. A. (2002). Church-based support groups for African American families coping with mental illness: Outreach and outcomes. *Journal of Psychiatric Rehabilitation, 26,* 173–180.

Pinquart, M., & Sorenson, S. (2005). Ethnic differences in stressors, resources, and psychological outcomes of family caregiving: A meta-analysis. *Gerontologist, 45,* 90–106.

Rozario, P. A., & DeRienzis, D. (2008). Familism, beliefs and psychological distress among African American women caregivers. *Gerontologist, 48,* 772–780.

Salimbene, S. (2000). *What language does your patient hurt in? A practical guide to culturally competent patient care.* Amherst, MA: Diversity Resources.

Scharlach, A. E., Kellam, R., Ong, N., Baskin, A., Goldstein, C., & Fox, P. J. (2006). Cultural attitudes and caregiver service use: Lessons from focus groups with racially and ethnically diverse family caregivers. *Journal of Gerontological Social Work, 47,* 133–156.

Sinunu, M., Yount, K. M., & El Afify, N. A. (2009). Informal and formal long term care for frail older adults in Cairo, Egypt: Family caregiving decisions in a context of social change. *Journal of Cross Cultural Gerontology, 24,* 63–76. doi:10.1007/s10823-008-9074-6

Soliman, H. H., & Almotgly, M. M. (2011). Psychosocial profile of people with AIDS and their caregivers in Egypt. *Psychological Reports, 108,* 883–892.

The Commonwealth Fund. (1999). *Informal caregiving.* Retrieved from http://www.commonwealthfund.org/~/media/files/publications/data brief/1999/may/informal-caregiving/caregiving_fact_sheet-pdf.pdf

Valle, R., Yamada, A. M., & Barrio, C. (2004). Ethnic differences in social network help-seeking strategies among Latino and Euro-American dementia caregivers. *Aging and Mental Health, 8,* 536–543.

Villa, M. L., Cueller, J., Gamel, N., & Yeo, G. (1993). *Aging and health: Hispanic American elders* (2nd ed.). Stanford, CA: Stanford Geriatric Education Center.

Yount, K. M., & Khadr, Z. (2008). Gender, social change, and living arrangements among older Egyptians during the 1990s. *Population Research and Policy Review, 27,* 201–225.

4

What Speech-Language Pathologists Should Know

Joan C. Payne

Acute and Chronic Adult-Onset Disorders

Advances in medical science and technology, wide distribution of public health information in major media outlets, and greater availability of preventive health care have helped to decrease adult mortality rates from strokes, dementia, AIDS, some forms of cancer, and other debilitating conditions over the last two decades. Although health disparities in the United States have mitigated against positive health outcomes for all persons (Payne, 2014), more persons are living longer with chronic and acute conditions, but often with disorders of motor, cognitive, swallowing, speech, and language skills. These findings underscore the critical role that family caregivers play in assisting those with impaired communication and swallowing.

More than one million adults in the United States are diagnosed annually with a chronic brain disease or disorder. The need for both long-term care and support for family caregivers is dramatic. Many of these conditions, for example, dementia, stroke, and Parkinson's disease, are associated with increasing age. Given the aging of the U.S. population, it is expected that the incidence of these disorders will increase proportionately in the coming decades.

Adult brain-based disorders are of particular concern. The following adult-onset brain disorders have high incidence figures among adults: Alzheimer's disease (AD) and other forms of dementia, amyotrophic lateral sclerosis (ALS), brain tumors, epilepsy, HIV/AIDS, multiple sclerosis (MS), Parkinson's disease (PD), cerebrovascular accidents (CVAs), and traumatic brain injury (TBI). Annual incidence data for the United States are shown in Table 4–1 and Figure 4–1. These brain disorders have a significant impact on speech, swallowing, voice, language, and cognition. Although not as prevalent as the disorders shown

Table 4–1. Annual Incidence Data on Adult-Onset Brain-Based Disorders and Conditions

Diagnosis/Cause	People Diagnosed Annually
Alzheimer's Disease	250,000
Amyotrophic Lateral Sclerosis	5,000
Brain Tumor	33,039
Epilepsy	135,500
HIV (AIDS) Dementia	1,196
Multiple Sclerosis	10,400
Parkinson's Disease	54,927
Stroke	600,000
Traumatic Brain Injury	80,000
TOTAL ESTIMATED INCIDENCE	**1,170,062**

Source: Family Caregiver Alliance, National Center on Caregiving (2001). *Incidence and Prevalence of the Major Causes of Brain Impairment.* Retrieved from https://www.caregiver.org/incidence-and-prevalence-major-causes-brain-impairment. Permission to republish granted.

American Adults Affected

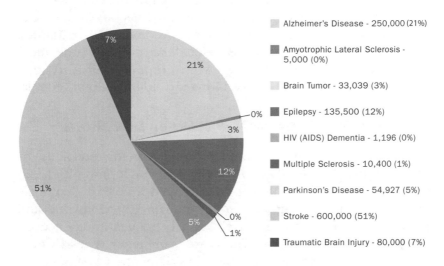

Figure 4–1. Annual prevalence of brain-based disorders among U.S. adults. Adapted from Family Caregivers Alliance National Center on Caregiving (2001).

in Table 4–1, other chronic conditions that can disrupt speech, language, voice, cognition, and swallowing in adults include progressive neuromotor disorders, such as adult-onset polio and myasthenia gravis, as well as adult intellectual disabilities, laryngeal cancer, and addictions.

When caring for adult brain-based acute and chronic disorders, caregivers must cope with changes in behavior, physical ability, stamina, and psychological disorders as well as limitations imposed by functional impairments. As disabled adults need around-the-clock care, several family members and friends from different households may be needed to become involved in the caregiving process (LaPointe, Murdoch, & Stierwalt, 2010).

Types of Brain-Based Disorders

There are several texts on adult brain-based disorders and diseases that provide comprehensive descriptions of their effects on communication and swallowing (Bayles & Tomoeda, 2013a, 2013b; Duffy, 2013; Freed, 2012; Hegde & Freed, 2011; LaPointe et al., 2010; Murray & Clark, 2015; Papathanasiou, Coppens, & Potagas, 2013; Payne, 2014; Swanepoel & Louw, 2010; Tanner, 2008). The following provides brief descriptions of the most prevalent brain-based disorders with emphases on caregiver reactions to communication, swallowing, and behavioral sequela.

Alzheimer's Disease (AD) and Other Dementias

Dementia is a progressive and rapidly growing problem for older adults. Deterioration of intellectual functioning and language makes this problem particularly difficult to diagnose. Dementia is now recognized as a syndrome of behavioral and personality characteristics, physiological changes, and effects on intelligence and cognition. There are four major types of neurodegenerative dementias: Alzheimer's dementia (AD), vascular dementia (VaD), Lewy-body dementia (LBD), and frontotemporal dementia (FTD). AD accounts for approximately 60% of all dementias and is the most well-known type. VaD, LBD, and FTD account for the remaining 40% of cases (Ripich & Horner, 2004). Of these irreversible dementias, AD, FTD, and VaD are the most prevalent and frequently coexist.

Alzheimer's Disease (AD). It is estimated that 5.4 million adults in the United States were diagnosed with AD in 2012, making it the most prevalence cause of dementia in aging adults (Alzheimer's Association, 2009; 2014a), followed by VaD. New drug treatments, such as Aricept, Razadyne, Namenda, Excelon, and Cognex, have lengthened the functional memories of persons with AD enabling them to live in the community for longer periods of time than in past decades. Table 4–2 gives the drug and brand names of drugs, AD stage, and FDA date of approvals.

Both language and cognition are affected by AD and VaD but in different ways. In AD, semantic retrieval and memory are affected. Semantic memory is responsible for categorization, visual memory, and the conceptualization of steps necessary to prepare a meal, get ready for bed, or plan a family reunion. This ability to conceptualize and order associated concepts and

Table 4–2. FDA-Approved Drug Treatments for Alzheimer's Disease

Drug Name	Brand Name	Approved for	FDA Approved
1. Donepezil	Aricept	All stages	1996
2. Galantamine	Razadyne	Mild to moderate	2001
3. Memantine	Namenda	Moderate to severe	2003
4. Rivastigmine	Exelon	Mild to moderate	2000
5. Tacrine	Cognex	Mild to moderate	1993

Source: Retrieved from http://www.alz.org/research/science/alzheimers_disease _treatments.asp

proposition is what Bayles (1988) refers to as a schema. In AD, also, there are three documented stages of the disease, ranging from mild to severe. Persons with AD tend to compensate for their loss of words in the mild stage, but in the moderate stage, naming errors, discourse incoherence, inability to answer questions, difficulty with automatic speech, and limitations in writing are obvious.

Vascular Dementia (VaD). Vascular dementia is the loss of intellectual functioning because of significant cerebrovascular disease and repeated strokes (Payne, 2014). VaD is a mixed dementia with both cortical and subcortical involvement. Persons with this dementia are more heterogeneous in their signs and symptoms than persons with AD and display a wider variety of symptoms. Clinical symptoms vary because of differences in locus of pathology.

Most persons with VaD are younger than persons with AD and have a history of hypertension and a fluctuating disease course. There is usually a history of previous strokes, abrupt onset of mental deterioration, and a stepwise course of "patchy" losses of functioning which lead to an uneven and erratic decline in functioning (Payne, 2014). In addition, persons with VaD are depressed and emotionally labile and frequently present with somatic complaints and focal neurologic signs.

Depending on the site of lesion in VaD, language disorders can include aphasia, visual agnosia and inability to recognize faces, anomia, and alexia with agraphia. Speech disorders include apraxia, emotionally toned speech disorder, dysarthria, and dysphagia. Cognitive disorders include decreased initiative and disturbances of motivation, dementia, and memory (Payne, 2014).

Frontotemporal Dementia (FTD). FTD, which includes Pick's disease, is characterized by progressive, fluent, empty speech, loss of word meaning, and semantic paraphasic errors (Bayles & Tomoeda, 2007). FTD is a complex dementia that includes a behavioral variant (bvFTD) subgroup. Persons with bvFTD display behaviors that are either impulsive (disinhibited) or bored and lethargic. Other behavioral changes are decreased insight, distractibility, an unusual interest in sex, changes in food preferences, neglect of personal hygiene, repetitive or compulsive behaviors, and blunted interest in personal relations and social life (NINDS, 2012). Mixed dementias, characterized by symptoms of AD and another type of dementia, are thought to be more pervasive than previously thought (Alzheimer's Association, 2014a).

Lewy Body Dementia (LBD). LBD has several symptoms that are associated with AD, but it is characterized by more severe deficits in verbal fluency and executive functioning. An important defining feature of LBD is a fluctuation in cognitive signs which is not found in PD or AD. The presence of abnormal motor behaviors in LBD makes it difficult to distinguish from PD. As the disease progresses, behavioral problems and dementia develop (Alzheimer's Association, 2014b).

Caregiver Reactions. Caregiving for a person with dementia can be extremely stressful and demanding. At the moderate stage, family members often become alarmed enough to seek medical attention and a diagnosis. The most commonly identified stressors for caregivers of persons with AD were memory deficits, loss of ability to communicate, and the gradual decline of intellect and personality of a loved one (Williamson & Schulz, 1993), although patterns of coping with these stressors varied depending on the social contacts or outlets of the caregivers (Lin & Hseuh-Sheng, 2014).

Vetter and colleagues (1999) observed a relationship between stages of severity in AD and VaD and caregiver burden. In early stage AD and VaD, caregivers of persons with VaD reported that patients imposed a greater burden on family caregivers than did persons with AD. In severe stage AD and VaD, this relationship underwent a reversal, with family caregivers of persons with AD experiencing the burden more adversely than those of persons with VaD.

Perhaps the most stressful type of dementia is FTD, particularly the behavioral variant subtype. Unlike AD, FTD presents with significant behavioral changes, making it a more difficult dementia for caregivers to manage. FTD patients are more affected in terms of dementia symptoms, and in congruence with the literature, FTD patients have more aberrant motor behaviors, disinhibition, apathy, and euphoria, whereas AD patients suffer significantly more from depressive symptoms (Riedijk et al., 2006).

Caregivers of persons with LBD report moderate to severe burden, Results of a Web-based survey to 962 caregivers of persons with LBD indicated that 80% felt the people around them did not understand their burden, and 54% reported feelings of isolation. Spousal caregivers reported more burden than did nonspousal caregivers. These caregivers also reported that the most common initial symptoms were cognitive (48%), motor (39%), or both (13%). Caregivers expressed concerns about fear of future (77%), feeling stressed (54%), loss of social life (52%), and uncertainty about what to do next (50%). Only 29% hired in-home assistance, whereas less than 40% used respite or adult day care, geriatric case managers, or attended a support group meeting. Lack of service utilization occurred despite two thirds of caregivers reporting medical crises requiring emergency services, psychiatric care, or law enforcement (Galvin et al., 2010).

Amyotrophic Lateral Sclerosis (ALS)

In ALS, nerve cells (neurons) waste away or die and can no longer send messages to muscles. This eventually leads to muscle weakening, twitching, and an inability to move the arms, legs, and body. The condition gradually gets worse. When the muscles in the chest area stop working, it becomes hard or impossible to breathe on one's own. Over time, people with ALS progressively lose the ability to function and care for themselves (Rowland & Shneider, 2001). Death often occurs within 3 to 5 years of diagnosis. About 25% of patients survive for more than 5 years after diagnosis (Radunovic, Annane, Jewitt, & Mustfa, 2009).

Verbal fluency in adults with ALS may be impaired and may result from a higher-order dysfunction, which suggests that there are deficits in the attentional system or central executive component of working memory (Abrahams et al., 2000). Selective cognitive impairment in the form of verbal fluency deficits, most likely indicating executive dysfunction, appears relatively early on in the course of the disease, although language functions may become vulnerable as the disease progresses (Irwin, Lippa, & Swearer, 2007).

Caregiver Reactions.   More involved respiratory-impaired ALS patients are described by their caregivers as having clinically significant impairments in executive functioning (Strutt et al., 2012). Progressive, physically disabling conditions like PD, multiple sclerosis, and ALS impose a different strain on caregivers who are providing care in the face of a visibly wasting disease. Gauthier and his associates (2007) noted that ALS caregivers re-port more depression as time passes whereas their care recipients report less depression. This finding, it is posited, may be attributable to the patient's acceptance of the inevitability of the disease, or to cognitive decline, while their caregivers experienced grief and depression as the disease progressed. As the physical demands increase in ALS, so does caregiver depression which is worsened in some instances by hurt from perceived lack of appreciation for their care (Rabkin, Albert, Rowland, & Mitsumoto, 2009).

Brain Tumors

In 2000, more than 359,000 persons were living with a diagnosis of primary brain and CNS tumors in the United States (Davis, Kupelian, Freels, McCarthy, & Surawicz, 2001). Cancer-related aphasia is secondary to primary brain tumors, typically gliomas which come from glial cells, or the non-neuronal supportive tissue in the central nervous system. Brain tumors may cause a variety of neurological disorders, including aphasia. Approximately 30% to 50% of patients with primary brain tumors experience aphasia, and anomic aphasia is the primary symptom. Brain tumor-related aphasia is generally transient, but if the tumor is inoperable or recurrent, symptoms may continue to develop and worsen as time goes on (Shafi & Carozza, 2012).

New research on cancer patients describes a phenomenon called "chemo brain" that has been experienced during chemotherapy by some patients who describe it as a state of cognitive decline (Asher, 2011). Although the brain usually recovers, some mental changes experienced by patients with cancer might last for a short period of time, or the changes may persist for years. Those affected may be unable to return to school, work, or social activities, or may find it difficult to return to daily activities.

A noncancerous (benign) tumor is the acoustic neuroma. Acoustic neuromas are usually slow-growing tumors that develop on the main nerve leading from the inner ear to the brain. Because branches of this nerve directly influence balance and hearing, pressure from an acoustic neuroma can cause hearing loss, ringing in the ear, and unsteadiness (Perry, Gantz, & Rubenstein, 2001). Also known as vestibular schwannoma, acoustic neuroma is an uncommon cause of hearing loss. An acoustic neuroma usually grows slowly or not at all, but in a few cases it may grow rapidly and become large enough to press against the brain and interfere with vital functions. Treatments for acoustic neuroma include regular monitoring, radiation, and surgical removal (Hain, 2012).

Caregiver Reactions. The diagnosis of a brain tumor is often made after a neurological episode that alerts medical specialists to look further for causes. The effect of the diagnosis on family members can be catastrophic. Family caregivers report high levels of stress, deteriorating physical and emotional health, career sacrifices, financial losses, and workplace discrimination. In addition, caregivers report that they must cope with cognitive impairment, seizures, and permanent neurological damage that may result from the disease or from treatments for the disease (Davis et al., 2001; Schubart, Kinzie, & Farace, 2008).

Epilepsy

Epilepsy can exist as an independent disorder or can coexist with AD (Halop, & Mucke, 2009). In AD, there is an increased incidence of unprovoked seizures possibly caused by high levels of β-amyloid peptides. Incidence of amnestic wandering has also been observed in persons with AD who have concurrent epilepsy (Hermann & Seidenberg, 2007).

Another type of epilepsy is refractory epilepsy which is epilepsy for which seizures are frequent and severe enough, or the required therapy for them is troublesome enough, to seriously interfere with quality of life (Epilepsy Foundation, 2014). Persons with refractory epilepsy report difficulty with memory, concentration and thinking, depression, and lethargy (Wheless, 2006).

Caregiver Reactions. Medication side effects are often difficult to manage and reduce quality of life (QOL) for caregivers significantly. Caregivers report that many of the negative consequences associated with epilepsy tend to be greater among those experiencing treatment side effects and a greater number of seizures (Wheless, 2006). Although persons with refractory epilepsy are much younger than persons with strokes or dementia, caregivers also report that their burden is similar to that of other neurological disorders in older adults. Furthermore, higher number of antiepileptic drugs, poorer patient neuropsychological performance, lower patient QOL score, and lower caregiver education level were associated with higher caregiver burden (Karakis et al., 2014).

HIV/AIDS

Chronic conditions resulting from positive HIV and AIDS status have become concerns for persons over age 50 (Wooten-Bielski, 1999). Currently, 1.1 million adults and adolescents are living with human immunodeficiency virus (HIV) infection in the United States, with 48,200 to 64,500 persons newly infected each year. HIV surveillance data show that 11% of all new AIDS cases are being diagnosed in mature adults aged 50 and older. Recent studies confirm that older adults are now contracting

HIV from intravenous drug use as well as from sexual contact. Statistics also show that new AIDS cases rose faster in the over-50 population than in people under 40. People aged 55 and older accounted for almost one-fifth (19%, or 217,000) of the estimated 1.1 million people living with HIV infection in the United States in 2010 (CDC, 2013).

Given the new drug therapies, however, mature adults who contract HIV can expect to live a normal life span. However, this group is vulnerable to strokes and dementia from opportunistic infections in the cerebral cortex and underlying white matter (Cole et al., 2004). Mizusawa, Hirano, Llena, and Shintaku (1988) found that cerebrovascular lesions associated with asymptomatic AIDS were found in 28 of 53 cases studied. Large cerebral infarcts were not clinically evident for most of the subjects. Rather the infarcts were small, multiple lesions that primarily involved the basal ganglia, cerebral cortex, and brainstem. Significant and pathologic changes in the blood vessels associated with the disease were suggested as possible causes (Mizusawa et al., 1988).

Patients with HIV-associated dementia complex (HAD) frequently develop focal lesions and language disorders as the disease progresses (Harezlak et al., 2011). Patients may exhibit difficulty with understanding spoken words as well as a tendency to misinterpret or mishear what is said. Expressive language problems can also occur, such as word-finding difficulties and slowed or slurred speech. At the end stage, mutism and nonresponsiveness may occur (Boccellari & Zeifert, 1994). Other symptoms include memory loss that is related to cortical atrophy (McArthur et al., 1993). Additional impairments include hearing loss, impaired respiratory functioning that affects vocal quality, major cognitive dysfunction in younger adults, and swallowing disorders (McNeilly, 2010).

Caregiver Reactions. Turner and Catania (1997) found that the largest group of caregivers to persons with AIDS (PWAs) are male friends—a group not typically found among caregivers to persons with other types of illnesses. Those reporting the greatest caregiver burden are gay or bisexual caregivers, caregivers who have traditional family ties to the PWA, men relative to women, and lower-income caregivers. The extent of caregiver burden from caring for a person who is HIV-positive or who has AIDS is explained by the Center for AIDS Prevention Studies:

> Many caregivers of AIDS patients are also their sexual partners. This puts them at risk for HIV infection. For HIV-positive caregivers, disease progression symbolizes the loss of their partner as well as their own changing health status. Caregiving also raises the question of who will care for them when they become ill. Informal caregivers may experience numbness, compassion fatigue, or burnout from losing multiple friends and loved ones to AIDS, or from caring for someone who has been ill for a very long time. In some communities there is still fear and stigma surrounding HIV disease. In addition, people greatly affected by AIDS are often already stigmatized populations: gay men, injection drug users, African-Americans and Latinos. Caregivers may fear social rejection, loss of job and/or housing and may thus conceal their caregiving status from family, friends, and co-workers. (Center for AIDS Prevention Studies, 1996)

Multiple Sclerosis (MS)

MS is an autoimmune disease frequently diagnosed in adults between 20 and 40 years of age. However, adults of any age can develop this disorder. MS causes motor disorders, specifically speech and swallowing disorders, because of destruction of the myelin sheath from inflammation which slows synaptic transmission from one neuron to another (National Multiple Sclerosis Society, 2008).

This disease has a variable course that affects each person differently. MS symptoms can vary because the location and severity of each attack can be different. Episodes can last for days, weeks, or months. These episodes alternate with periods of remission (Calabresi, 2007). Persons with MS complain of weakness, lack of coordination, and impaired vision and speech (Bear, Connors, & Paradiso, 2001).

Four disease courses have been identified in MS: relapsing-remitting MS (RRMS), primary-progressive MS (PPMS), secondary-progressive MS (SPMS), and progressive-relapsing MS. Each of these disease courses might be mild, moderate, or severe (Lublin & Reingold, 1996)

Relapsing-Remitting MS (RRMS). RRMS is the most common disease course and is characterized by clearly defined attacks of worsening neurologic function. These attacks—also called relapses, flare-ups, or exacerbations—are followed by partial or complete recovery periods (remissions), during which symptoms improve partially or completely and there is no apparent progression of disease. Approximately 85% of people with MS are initially diagnosed with RRMS.

Secondary-Progressive MS (SPMS). The name for this course comes from the fact that it follows after the relapsing-remitting course. Most people who are initially diagnosed with RRMS will eventually transition to SPMS, which means that the disease will begin to progress more steadily (although not necessarily more quickly), with or without relapses.

Primary-Progressive MS (PPMS). PPMS is characterized by steadily worsening neurologic function from the beginning. Although the rate of progression may vary over time with occasional plateaus and temporary, minor improvements, there are no distinct relapses or remissions. About 10% of people with MS are diagnosed with PPMS.

Progressive-Relapsing MS (PRMS). This is the least common of the four disease courses and is characterized by a steadily progressing disease process from the beginning with occasional exacerbations along the way. People with this form of MS may or may not experience some recovery following these attacks; the disease continues to progress without remissions.

Caregiver Reactions. MS is a variable disease with frequent bouts of hospitalizations and remissions. Figved, Myhr, Larsen, and Aarsland (2007) observed that the severity of caregiver burden was particularly high among spouses of persons with MS. The more the patient was physically impaired, the higher was the burden. Decreased cognition is common as is depression in MS, but the most disturbing behaviors to caregivers were patient delusions, disinhibition, agitation or aggressiveness, and irritability.

Depending on the course and severity of the disease, caregivers can feel increasingly overwhelmed. These perceptions can and do affect mental health status. Hillman (2013) reports that the average caregiver is a male in a spousal/partner relationship with a person with MS for many years who devotes 4 hours or more daily to care. The perception of burden has been found to be significantly greater among male caregivers than among female caregivers. Moreover, greater burden is associated with more frequent patient bladder dysfunction, more hours per week spent providing assistance, and greater restrictions on the caregiver's ability to perform daily activities because of caregiving responsibilities (Buchanan, Radin, & Huang, 2011).

Parkinson's Disease (PD)

PD is the most common of the age-related diseases of the basal ganglia and affects 1.5 million adults in the United States. Non-Hispanic whites have a substantially higher prevalence of PD than African or Asian Americans, and there may be a "Parkinson disease belt" in the Midwest and Northeast regions (Wright Willis, Evanoff, Lian, Criswell, & Racette, 2010).

The disease has no known etiology and is caused by insufficient dopamine in the basal ganglia. PD is a progressive motor disease that can present solely as a motor disorder or as a motor disorder that also affects cognition or speech fluency. As PD progresses, it often results in a severe dementia similar to LBD or AD (Alzheimer's Association, 2014b). Depression is a major problem in PD and is thought to occur in 40% of persons diagnosed. Depression may be associated with changes in cerebrospinal levels, a past history of depression, greater functional disability, greater left brain involvement, female gender, and early age at disease onset (Cummings, 1992). Approximately half of depressed patients with PD meet criteria for major depressive episodes. Remy, Doder, Lees, Turianski, and Brooks (2005) observed that depression in PD may be associated also with a specific loss of dopamine and noradrenaline innervation of cortical and subcortical components of the limbic system. The limbic system is responsible for instinctual and affective behavior and auditory memory.

There are four categories of possible etiologies for PD: idiopathic or unknown etiology, drug induced, postencephalitic causes from encephalitis or influenza, and arteriosclerotic PD associated with cerebral arteriosclerosis. Idiopathic PD, or PD of unknown etiology, accounts for the majority of the causes. Drug-induced PD is the second most common type (Brigo, Erro, Marangi, Bhatia, & Tinazzi, 2014). Medical advances in drug therapies or surgical intervention for some Parkinson's patients may forestall the worst symptoms, but there are no cures for this disease.

Caregiver Reactions. Aarsland, Larsen, Karlsen, Lim, and Tandberg (1999) found that caring for a spouse with PD is associated with emotional and social distress. Quality of the spousal relationship before a diagnosis of PD is an indicator of how caregivers perceive their level of burden. Caregiver distress increases if spousal caregivers feel that the marital relationship was unhappy before the disease occurred. Also, older age and gender may influence the extent of caregiver burden. Women and older caregivers report more stress than men and younger caregivers of persons with PD (Morley et al., 2012).

Cognitive and behavioral problems associated with PD are particularly stressful. Caregivers report an increase in their caregiver burden as the disease progresses in disability and PD symptoms, such as depression, hallucinations, confusion, and falls, emerge (Schrag, Hovris, Morley, Quinn, & Jahanshahi, 2006).

Cerebrovascular Accident (CVA) or Stroke

Each year, approximately 600,000 to 795,000 persons suffer a new or recurring CVA. From 1997 to 2007, the annual stroke death rate decreased by 34.3%, and the actual number of stroke deaths declined by 18.8%. The length of time to recover from a stroke depends on its severity.

Between 50% and 70% of persons who survive a CVA regain functional independence, but 15% to 30% are permanently disabled, and 20% require institutional care at 3 months after onset (American Heart Association, 2009). Among the community-living older adults examined by Kelly-Hayes and colleagues (2003), almost half (43%) of all persons with stroke had moderate to severe neurological deficits. Women were more dependent in

ADLs (33.9%) than men (15.6%). Women were less likely to walk unassisted (40.3% versus 17.8%) and more likely to live in nursing homes (34.9 % versus 13.3%). Older age accounted for the severity of disability. In this elderly cohort, more women experienced initial strokes and were more disabled at 6 months poststroke than did men. However, older age at stroke onset, not gender or stroke subtype, was associated with greater disability.

Data from the Acute Stroke Data Bank (Ramasubbu, Robinson, Flint, Kosier, & Price, 1998) show that some persons who survive stroke may have persistent aphasia, dysarthria, sensory deficits, visual field deficits (hemianopsia), and motor involvement after six or more months poststroke. Additional findings come from LaPointe and others (2010) who estimated that 1,079,000 persons in the United States have aphasia and from Code and Herrmann (2003) who posited that approximately 100,000 persons acquire aphasia each year.

Caregiver Reactions. After acute care and stroke rehabilitation, 80% of persons who survive a CVA return to the community, relying on their family members' emotional, informational, and instrumental support for daily living. Among the three (3) million stroke survivors in 1989, approximately 23% had VaD (American Heart Association, 2009). Caregivers of persons recovering from strokes have to cope with not only the survivors' difficulties with mobility and self-care, but also their aphasia, cognitive impairment, depression, and personality changes (Ross & Morris, 1988).

Family caregivers are mostly females who report that their life satisfaction is directly related to the severity of the stroke and the associated disabilities (Carod-Artal, Ferreira, Trizotto, & Menezes, 2009). Others report that their most important determinants of quality of life were their own age and their patient's functional status (Jönsson, Lindgren, Hallström, Norrving, & Lingren, 2005). For many, caregiving stress is directly related to the amount of time needed to assist in ADLs for those with limitations in mobility and independence. An additional source of caregiver stress is that many stroke survivors are unable to resume their prestroke occupations, a factor that increases financial strain for the family (Ellis, Dismuke, & Edwards, 2010; Jullamate, de Azeredo, Rosenberg, Pául, & Subgranon, 2007; Segal & Schall, 1996).

Families of persons who survive stroke may not feel that speech-language pathologists address their needs completely. In a study by Manders, Marien, and Janssen (2011), 77 family members (and 132 speech-language pathologists) were surveyed about the significance they attached to being informed, supported, and trained by speech-language pathologists. Speech-language pathologists were asked about the importance of informing and supporting family members and whether they felt that they provided adequate care in that area of need. Results showed that over 50% of all aspects concerning information and support were considered as (very) important by family members and SLPs alike. However, family members, and in particular, younger relatives, felt that speech-language pathologists did not meet some of the needs that they indicated were important.

Traumatic Brain Injury (TBI)

Older adults are among the most at-risk populations for TBIs from falls and pedestrian-related and vehicular accidents. Head injuries in this population can be most severe because of other complicating health problems that can interfere with memory, speech, swallowing, cognition, and hearing, making this group among those who will need long-term care and assistance from caregivers (Payne, Wright-Harp, & Davis, 2014)

Another population is that of armed services personnel deployed to war zones. Many returning veterans from the Desert Storm, Iraq, and Afghanistan conflicts have sustained life-threatening injuries. Multisystem and missile blast injuries that cause traumatic head injuries will require medical attention and family support for years to come (Okie, 2005). In particular, the nature of TBIs in this population will warrant long-term rehabilitation from speech-language pathologists (Cherney et al., 2010) and audiologists (Helfer et al., 2011). A number of communication and swallowing disorders from blast injuries, in isolation or in combination, have been reported by Wallace (2006) to be

- cognitive communication impairments related to traumatic brain injury (TBI),
- swallowing impairments,

- aphasia (due to stroke or focal traumatic brain injury),
- motor speech impairment,
- oral and facial burns or other trauma that impacts communication,
- smoke inhalation and resulting laryngeal trauma that impact communication,
- medical conditions requiring tracheotomies and ventilation, and
- hearing loss.

These communication and swallowing problems are complicated by the following (Payne, Wright-Harp, & Davis, 2014):

- Physically and emotionally traumatic circumstances and extreme environments in which many injuries are sustained
- Post-traumatic stress syndrome
- Multiple comorbidities (e.g., concomitant physical injuries to other parts of the body, seizures, pain, headaches, acoustic trauma, sensory impairments, depression, substance abuse)
- Possible repetitive and cumulative concussions sustained during combat duty

Caregiver Reactions. TBI is a catastrophic disorder for which most caregivers are ill prepared. Caregivers report differing symptoms of anxiety and depression at various stages after injury. Within 6 months after injury, a significant number of caregivers report clinically significant symptoms of anxiety and depression, and poor social adjustment. By 1 year postinjury, caregivers report that they are still depressed and anxious, but fewer caregivers report poor social adjustment. The initial impact on caregivers may be short-lived because caregivers have time to adapt and to learn some practical ways to manage the behavioral problems associated with TBI. However, persistent behavioral and cognitive problems increase the distress experienced by some caregivers over time. Further, caregiver burden is worsened by the social isolation demonstrated by the care recipient (Marsh, Kersel, Havill, & Sleigh, 2002).

Other Disabling or Chronic Conditions

Although not as prevalent as the brain-based disorders described earlier, the following disorders afflict mature adults and can impair speech, language, cognition, voice, or swallowing. These are chronic conditions that require care over time and can also cause high levels of anxiety and stress among caregivers.

Myasthenia Gravis

Myasthenia gravis is an autoimmune disease. An autoimmune disease causes the body to attack healthy tissue. In myasthenia gravis, the body produces antibodies that block the muscle cells from receiving messages from acetylcholine and other neurotransmitters on the postsynaptic side of the neuromuscular junction. This interference prevents the muscle contraction from occurring. Myasthenia gravis can affect people at any age, but it is most common in young women and older men. Prevalence of the disease is highest in elderly men.

A myasthenic crisis occurs when the muscles that control breathing weaken to the point that ventilation is inadequate, creating a medical emergency and requiring a respirator for assisted ventilation. In individuals whose respiratory muscles are weak, crises—which generally call for immediate medical attention—may be triggered by infection, fever, an adverse reaction to medication, or with under- or overuse of medication (NINDS, 2014). Crisis situations may occur without warning. These attacks seldom last longer than a few weeks. Hospitalization and assistance with breathing may be required during these attacks (Vincent & Newsom-Davis, 2007).

The cause of the disease is unknown, but it may result from tumors on the thymus gland (Vincent & Newsom-Davis, 2007). There is no cure for this disease, but medications and surgical removal of the thymus are documented to alleviate the severity of the symptoms.

Weakness of the voluntary (skeletal) muscles worsens with activity and improves with rest. Muscles needed to produce speech are significantly affected. One of the first symptoms is dysphonia (Montero-Odasso, 2006). Rare cases of dysphagia as the only initial symptom have also been reported (Romo González, Chaves, & Capello, 2010).

Post-Polio Syndrome (PPS)

PPS is the recurrence of polio in adults after remission in childhood. PPS is characterized by neurologic, musculoskeletal, and other general manifestations. Neurologic manifestations include new weakness, muscle atrophy, dysphagia, dysphonia, and respiratory failure. Musculoskeletal manifestations include muscle pain and joint pain. Other symptoms include generalized fatigue and cold intolerance. In a study of 350 adults diagnosed with post-polio syndrome, nearly 60% reported that the return of polio resulted in increased severity of disabilities and handicaps, particularly in the areas of occupation and social integration (Ivanyi et al., 1999).

There is no cure, but some medications and nonfatiguing exercises for mild-to-moderate new muscle weakness seem to help. Bulbar muscle weakness includes dysphagia, dysphonia, sleep disorders, and chronic respiratory failure. Dysphagia may be improved with instruction on compensatory swallowing techniques. Dysphonia is treated with voice exercise therapy and voice amplification devices (Jubelt, 2004).

Laryngeal Cancer

A laryngectomy is the removal of the larynx from the neck, usually because of cancer. During this operation, a new route for breathing is surgically created. The end of the trachea is connected to a stoma made in the neck which enables the person to breathe. Air inhaled into the lungs through the stoma is no longer warmed or moisturized by structures of the nose and mouth. As a result, the trachea can become irritated which creates a thick mucus. This mucus may also crust on the stoma and require routine removal. The patient may benefit from humidifiers and a cover to protect the stoma (ASHA, n.d.). Laryngectomized patients need to take special care in cleaning their stomas and must avoid heavy lifting.

In addition to learning to speak in a new way, persons with laryngectomies who are also undergoing chemotherapy may show signs of neoplastic aphasia and may need additional assistance to cope with the mental changes, such as forgetting names, memory lapses, and inability to multitask (Asher, 2011).

Intellectual Disabilities

Adults diagnosed in childhood with intellectual disabilities are living longer into middle age and integrating into communities. While some live in group homes or other sheltered living facilities, others live with their families. Two categories of adults are considered: those diagnosed with cerebral palsy and those diagnosed with Down syndrome. Adults with cerebral palsy do not always present with disabilities that impact intellectual functioning, however.

Adults with cerebral palsy may evidence drooling and swallowing disorders. In addition, recurrent infections because of aspiration and urinary incontinence may be problematic. Adults with Down syndrome present with a different clinical picture, including dementia after age 50, recurring cerumen impactions, and hearing loss (Prater & Zylstra, 2006).

Addictions

Although not typically thought of as diseases that compromise language or cognition, addictions to alcohol, illegal drugs like cocaine and methamphetamine, and prescription drugs have been found to be associated with strokes and significant cognitive changes. Even after the adult has received treatment for addictions, many functional problems persist.

The problem of drug addiction is more pervasive than originally thought. Rates of current illicit drug use among persons aged 50 to 64 increased from 2002 to 2012. Much of this increase is attributed to the aging of the baby boomer cohort (born between 1946 and 1964) into the 50 or older age group. This cohort, particularly those born after 1950, had much higher rates of illicit drug use as teenagers and young adults than older cohorts. This generational shift in drug use is still evident in the most recent data. The drugs consumed by older adults included marijuana and nonmedical use of prescription drugs, cocaine, heroin, hallucinogens, and inhalants (Substance Abuse and Mental Health Services Administration, 2013).

There is an underrepresentation of older adult alcoholics in the literature; however, the National Institute of Alcoholism and Alcohol Abuse (2012) reports that 15.3 million adults meet the criteria for an alcohol use disorder, and that of those, 2.3 million adults meet the criteria for a drug use disorder. Unfortunately, misuse and abuse of alcohol and other drugs take a greater toll on affected older adults than on younger adults. In addition to the psychosocial issues that are unique to older adults, aging ushers in biomedical changes that influence the effects that alcohol and drugs have on the body. Alcohol abuse, for example, may accelerate the normal decline in physiological functioning that occurs with age. In addition, alcohol may elevate older adults' high risk for injury, illness, and socioeconomic decline (Center for Substance Abuse Treatment, 1998).

Adults bound to their homes are at great risk for alcoholism. Persons who are homebound because of other health problems, such as heart problems, diabetes, chronic lung diseases, and other conditions, are often limited in their mobility. These conditions diminish the adult's ability to perform the basic tasks of daily living and increase the reliance on caregivers. Chronic alcohol abuse may result, also, in a form of dementia, called Korsakoff's disease (KD) which is characterized by generalized cortical atrophy. The cognitive changes associated with KD develop as a secondary dementia and occur after long-term alcohol abuse and vitamin B deficiency. Symptoms of the dementia are mild and either nonprogressive or slowly progressive (Payne, 2014).

Cocaine-induced strokes have been reported for adults in their middle years. This applies to both the powdered and crack cocaine (Wallace, 1993). Stroke severity has been related to long-term effects of cocaine use, repeated strokes, and other neuropathies associated with being a polydrug user (Payne, 2014). Other drugs of choice that are typically used in addition to cocaine are alcohol, marijuana, heroin, and nicotine (Brown, Serganian, & Tremblay, 1994). There is a high prevalence of psychiatric disorders, particularly depression, in older adults and a known link with drug abuse. The overall trend is for a rise in the prevalence of cocaine use, and thus an expected similar rise in use by members of the older population is likely (Lofwall, Schuster, & Strain, 2008).

Summary

The average ages of persons who are care recipients range from 50 to 75 years of age. As adults age, there are a number of diseases and conditions that affect them and compromise all aspects of functional independence and communication, specifically, expressive and receptive language, motor speech, swallowing, verbal fluency, discourse, and pragmatics. Any one of the disorders described in this chapter can disrupt effective interactions between caregivers and their care recipients. However, there is frequently a combination of speech, language, voice, cognitive, or swallowing disorders that can negatively affect quality of life and make communication extremely frustrating for caregivers.

Consistent themes in how caregivers react to long-term caring for persons with brain-based disorders are high anxiety, depression, and poor physical and emotional health. Many of the brain-based disorders include behavioral and cognitive disorders that worsen the caregiver's ability to manage care.

The suddenness of acute disorders such as stroke and traumatic brain injury cause significant caregiver stress. Most caregivers are devastated and unprepared to deliver care unless educated and empowered to help their loved one.

Chronic disorders like dementia, MS, ALS, and AIDS involve long-term changes in personality, behavior, motor ability, and intellectual abilities. Other, less prevalent chronic disorders, such as myasthenia gravis, post-polio syndrome, adult developmental delays and addictions also compromise communication and swallowing and can impose caregiver stress and fatigue. Caring for persons with long-term chronic disorders involves major sacrifices in time, energy, and finances. These caregivers of disabled adults need education and resources to maintain a consistent level of care. Similarly, caregivers for persons diagnosed with cancer, whether brain or laryngeal cancer, need special consideration for caregiver distress and burnout.

Caregivers frequently complain that they do not understand medical jargon and, therefore, have little understanding of the implications of acute and chronic conditions for communication and swallowing. Some disorders that compromise language, speech, swallowing, voice, or cognition are the result of lifestyle, specifically pharmaceutical and illicit drug abuse and unprotected sexual activity, and should be discussed with caregivers in an open and sensitive manner. Sensitivity is also called for in educating caregivers about other diagnoses like dementia, stroke, head injuries, and progressive motor disorders. There are a variety of resources available for caregivers that provide easily understandable written and video materials about the acute and chronic disorders discussed in this chapter. See Table 4–3 for contact information and types of caregiver information available at each site. These resources can be shared in conjunction with other information given to help caregivers understand the nature of the disabilities, their relationship to communication disorders, and resources and self-care tips for family and friends who are providing care.

Helping the Caregiver to Avoid Communication Breakdowns

Speech-language pathologists can help to minimize some areas of caregiver stress, particularly in the areas of improving communication between caregivers and care recipients. One way is by providing assistance to the caregiver on how to improve interactions with an adult who has impaired communication. It is important that the caregiver feel supported and encouraged in carrying out this type of training with a loved one. For some caregivers, avoiding or repairing communication breakdowns may be extremely challenging to carry out. Compliance will be better if the speech-language pathologist regularly monitors how the caregiver is doing (Hilton & Leenhouts, 2014). Discussions can focus on (a) whether the caregiver feels that a particular strategy is working to improve communication, and (b) which alternative strategies should be considered if a strategy is less than successful. To help with these discussions, caregivers can make daily notations in a journal to share with the speech-language pathologist.

Table 4–3. Resources for Caregivers

Organization and Contact Details	Type of Information
Multiple Disorders Sites	
American Speech, Language Hearing Association http://www.asha.org 2200 Research Boulevard Rockville, MD 20850-3289 (800) 638-8255	Reader-friendly information on brain-based disorders, injuries, and cancer including descriptions, causes of disorders, effects on communication, and resources.
AARP http://www.aarp.org 601 E. Street, NW Washington, DC 20049 (888) 687-2277	Links to caregiving for a variety of health disorders. Includes blog on caregiver self-care and information on cultural diversity among caregivers.
Stroke and Aphasia	
Aphasia Hope Foundation http://www.aphasiahope.org PO Box 26304 Shawnee, KS (855) 764-4673	Has browsing posts for caregivers to share ideas. Also provides information from professionals on new research and therapies. Includes featured curricula for learning more about caring for stroke survivors.
National Stroke Association http://www.stroke.org 9707 E. Easter Lane, Ste. B Centennial, CO 80112 (800) 787-6537	Gives information on stroke symptoms and recovery. Provides printable caregiving guide and webinars.
American Heart Association http://www.heart.org 7272 Greenville Ave. Dallas, TX 75231 (800) 242-8721	Provides printable resources for caregivers of persons with strokes.
National Aphasia Association http://www.aphasia.org 350 Seventh Ave., Ste. 902 New York, NY 10001 (800) 922-4622	Promotes public awareness and understanding of aphasia and provides support to all persons with aphasia and their caregivers, including such topics as aphasia facts and therapy, and a guide to assistive technology.

continues

Table 4–3. *continued*

Organization and Contact Details	Type of Information
Dementia	
Alzheimer's Association http://www.alz.org 225 N. Michigan Ave., Fl. 17 Chicago, IL 60601 (800) 272-3900	Provides an interactive website for assessing caregiving stress and providing resources to address the areas of stress.
Alzheimer's Disease Education and Referral Center, National Institute on Aging http://www.alzheimers.org PO Box 8250 Silver Spring, MD 20907-8250 (800) 438-4380	Includes information about ongoing studies on Alzheimer's disease and other dementias.
Lewy Body Dementia Association http://www.lbda.org 912 Killian Hill Road, SW Lilburn, GA 30047 (800) 539-9767	Offers an LBD caregiver link, featuring "Lewy Buddies," a toll-free LBD caregiver link, and email support for caregivers to ask questions and get information.
Traumatic Brain Injury	
Brain Trauma Foundation http://www.braintrauma.org 7 World Trade Center, 34th Floor 250 Greenwich St. New York, NY 10007 (212) 772-0608	Provides a TBI glossary, coma and concussion checklists, a patient narrative, and a link to patient and family resources, including the Traumatic Brain Injury Survival Guide.
Brain Injury Association of America http://www.biausa.org 1608 Spring Hill Road, Ste. 110 Vienna, VA 22182 (800) 444-6443	Provides educational information on living with brain injury and includes color illustrations of the structures and functions of the brain for educational purposes.
Brain Tumors	
Acoustic Neuroma Association http://www.anausa.org 600 Peachtree Parkway, Ste. 108 Cumming, GA 30041 (877) 200-8211	This site has links for caregiver resources and strategies for coping.

Table 4–3. *continued*

Organization and Contact Details	Type of Information
Brain Tumors *continued*	
American Brain Tumor Association http://www.abta.org 8550 W. Bryn Mawr Ave., Ste. 5 Chicago, IL 60631 (800) 886-2282	Provides caregiver resources, including a handbook for caregivers of persons with brain tumors and a caregiver checklist to help with organizing time and assigning tasks to volunteers, family, and friends. Also has online resources that provide financial and transportation assistance.
National Brain Tumor Society http://www.braintumor.org 55 Chapel Street, Ste. 200 Newton, MA 02458 (617) 924-9997	Has a link to caregiver resources, including a publication, *Orientation to Caregiving*, and a publication on caring for the caregiver.
Amyotrophic Lateral Sclerosis	
Amyotrophic Lateral Sclerosis Association http://www.alsa.org 1275 K Street NW, Ste. 250 Washington, DC 20005 (202) 407-8580	Caregiver tips and hints and links to resource sites. Also, links to resource sites and information on respite care, coping with burnout, and caregiver testimonials.
Muscular Dystrophy Association http://www.mda.org 222 S. Riverside Plaza, Ste. 1500 Chicago, IL 60606 (800) 572-1717	Caregivers will find a link that provides information on self-care and stress reduction.
Parkinson's Disease	
National Parkinson Foundation http://www.parkinson.org 200 SE 1st Street, Ste. 800 Miami, FL 33131 (800) 473-4636	Site features tutorials on caregiving, library and local resources, and discussion groups and blogs.

continues

Table 4–3. *continued*

Organization and Contact Details	Type of Information
Epilepsy	
Epilepsy Foundation http://www.epilepsy.com 8301 Professional Place Landover, MD 20785-2353 (800) 332-1000	Provides information about support groups, information for veterans, transportation resources, and a 24/7 hotline.
Multiple Sclerosis	
The National Multiple Sclerosis Society Information Resource Center and Library http://www.nationalmssociety.org 1700 Owens Street, Ste. 190 San Francisco, CA 94158 (800) 344-4867	Links to "Family Matters" which includes downloadable information for caregivers and tips on finding support and assistance.
Myasthenia Gravis	
Myasthenia Gravis Foundation of America http://www.myasthenia.org 355 Lexington Ave., 15th Floor New York, NY 10017 (800) 541-5454	Features calendars of chapter meetings, information on support groups, financial resources, and free clinics.
Adult Developmental Disabilities/Mental Retardation	
American Association on Intellectual Developmental Disabilities http://www.aaidd.org 501 3rd Street NW, Ste. 200 Washington, DC 20001 (202) 387-1968	Provides webinars for caregivers on a variety of topics (e.g., promoting oral hygiene, end-of-life care, disabilities, and aging).
Addictions	
Caring, Inc. http://www.caring.com 2600 El Camino Road, Ste. 300 San Mateo, CA 94403 (800) 973-1540	Links to caregiver solution center, online support, and addiction support groups.

Table 4–3. *continued*

Organization and Contact Details	Type of Information
Addictions *continued*	
American Psychological Association http://www.apa.org 750 First Street NE Washington, DC 20002-4242 (800) 374-2721	Links to caregiver facts, caregiver briefcase, and resources. Links to practice section for professionals who assist caregivers. Discussion of types of addictions and impact on family members.
Laryngeal Cancer	
American Cancer Society http://www.cancer.org 250 Williams Street NW Atlanta, GA 30303 (800) 227-2345	This site has links to information about caregiving and online communities and support. Also has links to caregiver and patient checklists for difficulties with coping and distress.
International Association of Laryngectomees http://www.theial.com 925B Peachtree Street NE, Ste. 316 Atlanta, GA 30309 (866) 425-3678	Information on conferences and support groups.
National Cancer Institute http://www.cancer.gov 9609 Medical Center Drive Bethesda, MD 20892-9760 (800) 422-6237	Site contains links to a variety of caregiver publications and references for additional reading.
Swallowing Disorders	
National Foundation of Swallowing Disorders http://www.swallowingdisorder foundation.com PO Box 3725 Carmel, CA 93921 (415) 326-3673	Site provides information on support groups and educational webinars.

Cognitive-Communication Disorders Associated With Dementia and TBI

Both dementia and TBI produce cognitive-communication disorders because of the diffuse nature of brain damage. Cognitive-communication disorders are characterized by difficulty organizing words logically, decreased word fluency and lexical richness, impaired pragmatic skills, memory disorders, and poor discourse cohesion. Persons with dementia, for example, may speak less often and will have difficulty finding the right words or may use familiar words repeatedly. Nonverbal gestures may be used more often to replace intended words. These problems often cause breakdowns in caregiver/care recipient communication.

Although there are many strategies caregivers can use to avoid or repair communication breakdowns with adults who have cognitive-communication disorders (Table 4–4), some are more frequently used and viewed to be more successful than others. Small, Gutman, Makela, and Hillhouse (2003) found that caregivers report that they most frequently (a) do not interrupt, (b) eliminate distractions, (c) approach the individual slowly to begin communication, and (d) use one-question instruction. The results of their study showed that the most successful strategies for eliminating communication breakdowns were (a) eliminating distractions, (b) using simple sentences, and (c) using yes/no questions. The most ineffective strategy was speaking slowly because the individual was required to retain and process the incoming information.

In a similar study (Wilson, Rochon, Milhailidis, & Leonard, 2012), caregivers used a number of communication strategies most successfully during task activities. The successful strategies were (a) presenting one idea or direction at a time, (b) using closed-ended questions, and (c) paraphrasing repetitions. Effective nonverbal communication strategies were (a) using guided touch, (b) pointing to an object, (c) handing an object to the resident, and (d) demonstrating an action (Wilson et al., 2012).

Other suggestions for caregivers can be helpful in assisting them to work with the adult with a cognitive-communication disorder. Some suggestions are to train caregiving on how to

- develop memory wallets and scrapbooks of family photographs;

Table 4–4. Suggested Strategies for Caregivers to Avoid Communication Breakdowns With Adults With Cognitive-Communication Disorders

---

To become a better listener, the caregiver should

- Be patient and supportive.
- Offer comfort and assurance.
- Avoid being argumentative.
- Encourage nonverbal communication (e.g., pointing or gesturing).

To use nonverbal cues to maximize communication effectiveness, the caregiver should

- Use guided touch.
- Demonstrate an action.
- Point to an object.
- Hand an object to the person.
- Begin the task.

To become a better speaker, the caregiver should

- Simplify directions to one at a time.
- Use yes/no questions.
- Speak clearly.
- Patiently wait for a response.
- Repeat information or questions; if necessary, paraphrase.
- Turn questions into answers (e.g., "The bathroom is right here.").
- Eliminate distractions from the environment while speaking (e.g., telephone, television, music).
- Refer to the person by name.
- Modify the environment to encourage conversation (e.g., lighting that enables the listener to see the speaker's face).
- Wait to speak until eye contact has been established and maintained.
- Give verbal praise.
- Provide orientation information at the beginning of each conversation.
- Keep topics familiar and observable.
- Modify statements in the person's language.

Source: Alzheimer's Association (2014); Brush and Calkin (2008); Shekim (1990); Small, Gutman, Makela, and Hillhouse (2003); and Wilson, Rochon, Milhailidis, and Leonard (2012).

- engage in guided reminiscences about special events;
- label items used in daily hygiene or personal care;
- participate in meal preparation and cleanup;
- join in regular conversations with a trusted communication partner;
- use functional communication through scenarios such as banking, ordering from a menu, using maps, and preparing grocery lists;
- practice explaining meanings in proverbs, idioms, sarcasm, and humor; and
- reinforce reality through orientation exercises.

Computer Software and Low-Tech Augmentative and Alternative Communication for Cognitive-Communication Disorders

Family caregivers can be assisted to use both low- and high-tech augmentative and alternative communication devices (Bourgeois, Fried-Oken, & Rowland, 2010; Gentry, Wallace, Kvarfordt, & Lynch, 2008; Yasuda, Kuwabara, Kuwahara, Abe, & Tetsutani, 2009) and computer software (Archibald, Orange, & Jamieson, 2009; Fink, Brecher, Sobel, & Schwartz, 2005; Wertz & Katz, 2004). In this information age, computer software designed to provide therapy to persons with cognitive-language disorders has become available for clinicians and for patients and their family caregivers who are comfortable with using the computer. Online resources for computer software, cognitive stimulation, and games and crafts for persons with cognitive-communication disorders can be accessed at http://www.best-alzheimer's-prod ucts.com, where interactive games like Bingo and Smartbrain can be downloaded. Smartbrain is a computer-based game that provides stimulation in cognitive skills like attention and memory. The usefulness of this game with mild to moderately impaired persons with cognitive-language disorders has been corroborated by research findings (Sobel, 2001; Tarraga et al., 2006).

In addition to memory wallets and books, low-tech devices can be used to support memory and language. Videophone technology and face-to-face computer messaging (Skype) used in therapy can also be used by caregivers (Yasuda et al., 2009). Other devices include talking photo albums and personal digital assistants (PDAs) to support memory (Gentry et al., 2008). Yasuda and colleagues have reported success in reducing behavioral disturbances by using personalized reminiscence photo videos (personal photos with narration and background music) and videophone technology. It is anticipated that as more adults age, there will be an increase in the use and modification of computers, cell phones, PDAs, and other electronic devices to support memory (Gentry et al., 2008).

Digital voice output, which works well for persons with aphasia, has not been as successful with persons with dementia (Bourgeois et al., 2010). However, voice output as digital speech reminders for daily tasks for persons with dementia may help them remain independent for a longer time.

Aphasia

Caregivers can be assisted with using techniques that are in keeping with client-centered therapy in aphasia, specifically, conversation training, response elaboration training (RET), and Promoting Aphasics Communication Effectiveness (PACE). In each of these techniques, the caregiver functions as a conversational partner who accepts the message sent by the person with aphasia. In conversation training, the caregiver helps the person with aphasia select the appropriate word, use nonverbal communication, and apply the rules of conversation.

RET emphasizes the content of the response rather than the form. The caregiver and care recipient (partner) can select a conversation topic. The caregiver then provides a series of prompts and asks the partner to add on to his or her original productions, with the goal being to lengthen the number of utterances produced by the partner.

Allowing the person with aphasia to use any modality to communicate messages is the hallmark of PACE. The goal is to improve conversational skills. Both the caregiver and the person with aphasia take turns as message sender or receiver, promoting active participation in conversation.

Augmentative/Assistive Communication

There is consensus that with training and careful selection of appropriate devices, persons with aphasia will benefit from augmentative and assistive communication (AAC). Johnson and her associates (2008) examined abilities of three individuals with chronic nonfluent aphasia (NA) using a dynamic display AAC device to enhance communication. The device, Dialect with Speaking Dynamically Pro, was tailored to each participant's skill level using a treatment protocol adapted from Koul, Corwin, and Hayes (2005) in which the primary caregiver was the spouse. Participants with aphasia showed improvement in pretreatment and posttreatment measures for quality and effectiveness of communication, and two participants showed improved linguistic and cognitive functioning.

The use of computers in therapy serves the purpose of increasing frequency of therapy by allowing patients to practice specific exercises at home. Training families to use computer-assisted therapy can help people with aphasia retrieve certain parts of speech, such as the use of verbs, and can be used to provide an alternative system of communication for people who have difficulty with expressive language. Auditory discrimination software with training exercises can also help patients who have problems perceiving the difference between phonemes.

Commercially available programs like Lingraphica™ use a multimodal treatment approach. Persons with aphasia are reported to increase natural and expressive language with this program (Aftonomos, Appelbaum, & Steele, 1999; Aftonomos, Steele, & Wertz, 1997). Another commercially available computer software program is AphasiaMate™ (Archibald et al., 2009) which is a comprehensive computer-based language therapy program with eight modules of learning. Archibald and her colleagues (2009) found increased improvement in language and functional communication skills, particularly for persons with moderate to severe aphasia. Newer technologies, such as VAST™ (Video Assisted Speech Technology), has been shown to be affective with persons with apraxia and persons with Broca's aphasia (Williams, 2014). More on VAST™ can be accessed from http://www.speakinmotion.com. This technology can be used in the clinic, and caregivers can be trained to use this at home.

It will be important for the speech-language pathologist to help caregivers select the most appropriate devices and to train them on how to use them. It will be equally important to assist caregivers with determining costs and the means by which such devices can be purchased, whether through Medicaid, Medicare, or private insurances.

Disorders of Speech

A major goal for supporting family caregivers should be to assist them in how to increase speech intelligibility so that messages sent by a person with a disorder of speech are at an appropriate rate and volume to be better understood. Dysarthria is a multi-faceted problem involving all areas of speech production: phonation, resonance, prosody, articulation, and respiration (Freed, 2012). Caregivers should be instructed to do the following:

- Slow the rate of speech by helping the person to clap out an intended message; use a metronome to pace each word or practice speaking using earphones.
- Enable the speaker to have greater lung volume by positioning the person upright in a chair during conversation.
- Increase prosody by asking a question and have the person answer it while adding stress on key words to emphasize the meaning of the answer.
- Use blowing and sucking exercises to increase tongue and lip mobility.
- Increase loudness by cuing the patient to speak more loudly.

Assistive Devices

There are several companies, like Parrot™, who offer a full range of computer programs that provide practice in speech both in the clinical setting and at home. Caregivers can use these programs to work on specific targets from therapy. In addition, two types of AAC devices, mid-tech and high-tech, are appropriate for persons with impairments of speech who have little or no speech. Mid-tech tools use prerecorded words or phrases and a button for each. The high-tech device has a keyboard, display, and speaker. Users type words that show up on the display and are spoken aloud by a computer voice. High-tech tools also have a screen that shows an array of buttons or a picture with "hotspots." Users press these buttons or hotspots to select a word or phrase, or to change the screen to a new set of choices. This gives people rapid access to a large vocabulary. The device speaks completed messages with very human sounding computer voices or recorded voices. These devices can be accessed by touch, gaze, or hitting switches with other parts of the body. They can also often be used to control devices such as lights or the television, or to control a computer.

Persons coping with progressive diseases like ALS may benefit from assistive devices that do not depend on muscular strength or speech to use. Tobii™, for example, has developed assistive technology devices that help those affected by ALS to regain and retain their independence. These devices can help with controlling the TV and DVD player and enable communication by phone, e-mail, and the Web. More advanced assistive devices can provide persons who have motor impairments with a voice. An additional eye-controlled device allows persons with progressive neurological disabilities to continue to communicate with family, friends, and doctors (Geronimo, Stephens, Schiff, & Simmons, 2014).

Assisting the Patient With Swallowing Disorders

Swallowing disorders present a physical threat to the adult, particularly if the adult has brain-based disorders. Caregivers will need assistance in reinforcing therapy goals and in identifying which foods are the most bothersome to swallow. Cooke (2008) also suggests that caregivers should (a) engage the person in decision making about meal choices; (b) make mealtime more of a social event; (c) avoid placing pressure to eat or drink; and (d) eat with the person, emulating some of the techniques used to facilitate swallowing. Some suggestions are to instruct caregivers to do the following:

- Set a tone of support and encouragement.
- Prepare colorful, culturally familiar, and appetizing foods to encourage eating. This is particularly helpful when the person is on a pureed diet.

- Encourage the use of head placements, such as turning the head to one side, to facilitate a better swallow.
- Encourage the person to sit up straight any time he or she eats or drinks and make sure all food is cleared from the mouth.
- Make mealtimes enjoyable, festive, and leisurely.
- Promote small bites and sips to avoid choking.
- Thicken liquids to decrease the possibility of choking.
- Exercise patience and give positive feedback.

Summary

Speech-language pathologists serve the important function of assisting family caregivers to communicate more effectively and facilitate safe swallowing habits for their loved ones. Caregivers can be trained by the speech-language pathologist to provide stimulating activities, engage in constructive conversations, use modified treatment techniques to improve speech and swallowing, and use assistive devices to complement or replace speech.

Ensuring that the caregiver is able to comply with training is a factor of establishing trust. Caregivers need to feel that they have the support and encouragement of the speech-language pathologist. Regular monitoring of how the caregiver is doing, being available for questions, and providing time for the caregiver to share perceptions of successes and failures of their approaches also help to establish and maintain compliance.

References

Aarsland, D., Larsen, J. P., Karlsen, K., Lim, N. G., & Tandberg, E. (1999). Mental symptoms in Parkinson's disease are important contributors to caregiver distress. *International Journal of Geriatric Psychiatry, 14*, 866–874.

Abrahams, S., Leigh, P. N., Harvey, A., Vythelingum, G. N., Grise, D., & Goldstein, L. H. (2000). Verbal fluency and executive dysfunction in amyotrophic lateral sclerosis (ALS). *Neuropsychologia, 38*, 734–747.

Aftonomos, L. B., Appelbaum, J. S., & Steele, R. D. (1999). Improving outcomes for persons with aphasia in advanced community-based treatment programs. *Stroke, 30*, 1370–1379.

Aftonomos, L. B., Steele, R. D., & Wertz, R. T. (1997). Promoting recovery in chronic aphasia with an interactive technology. *Archives of Physical Medicine and Rehabilitation, 78*, 841–846.

Alzheimer's Association. (2009). *Alzheimer's disease facts and figures.* Retrieved from http://www.alz.org/national/documents/report_alz factsfigures2009.pdf

Alzheimer's Association. (2014a). 2014 Alzheimer's disease facts and figures. *Alzheimer and Dementia: The Journal of the Alzheimer's Association, 10*, e47–e92. Retrieved from http://www.alzheimersand dementia.com/article/S1552-5260(14)000624/abstract

Alzheimer's Association. (2014b). *Current Alzheimer's treatments.* Retrieved from http://www.alz.org/research/science/alzheimers_ disease_treatments.asp?gclid=Cj0KEQjw6deeBRCswoauquC8haUB EiQAdq5zh9h-s_AUebOnSjRS7WSgMo0JCIpWsGu4BVmh2LTw430a AqlR8P8HAQ#approved

American Heart Association. (2009). AHA statistical update. Heart disease and stroke statistics 2009 update. *Circulation, 119*, e21–e181. doi:10.1161/CIRCULATIONAHA.108.191261

American Speech-Language-Hearing Association. (n.d.). *Laryngeal cancer.* Retrieved from http://www.asha.org/public/speech/disorders/ LaryngealCancer/

Archibald, L. M. D., Orange, J. B., & Jamieson, D. J. (2009). Implementation of computer-based language therapy in aphasia. *Therapeutic Advances in Neurologic Disorders, 2*, 299–311.

Asher, A. (2011). Cognitive dysfunction among cancer survivors. *American Journal of Physical Medicine and Rehabilitation, 90* (5 Suppl. 1), S16–S26.

Bayles, K. A. (1988). Language and dementia. In A. L. Holland (Ed.), *Language disorders in adults: Recent advances* (pp. 209–243). San Diego, CA: College-Hill Press.

Bayles, K. A., & Tomoeda, C. K. (2007). *Cognitive-communication disorders of dementia.* San Diego, CA: Plural.

Bayles, K. A., & Tomoeda, C. K. (2013a). *Cognitive-communication disorders of dementia* (2nd ed., pp. 123–158). San Diego, CA: Plural.

Bayles, K. A., & Tomoeda, C. K. (2013b). *MCI and Alzheimer's dementia: Clinical essentials for assessment and treatment of cognitive-communication disorders.* San Diego, CA: Plural.

Bear, M. F., Connors, B. W., & Paradiso, M. A. (2001). *Neuroscience: Exploring the brain* (2nd ed., pp. 613–615). Philadelphia, PA: Lippincott Williams & Wilkins.

Boccellari, A., & Zeifert, P. (1994). Management of neurobehavioral impairment in HIV-1 infection. *Psychiatric Clinics of North America: Psychiatric Manifestations of HIV Disease, 17,* 183–204.

Bourgeois, M., Fried-Oken, M., & Rowland, C. (2010, March 16). AAC strategies and tools for persons with dementia. *The ASHA Leader.*

Brigo, F., Erro, R., Marangi, A., Bhatia, K., & Tinazzi, M. (2014). Differentiating drug-induced parkinsonism from Parkinson's disease: an update on non-motor symptoms and investigations. *Parkinsonism and Related Disorders, 20,* 808–814. doi: 10.1016/j.park reldis.2014.05.011

Brodaty, H., & Donkin, M. (2009). Family caregivers of people with dementia. *Dialogues in Clinical Neuroscience, 11,* 217–228.

Brown, T. G., Serganian, P., & Tremblay, J. (1994). Alcoholics also dependent on cocaine in treatment: Do they differ from pure alcoholics? *Addictive Behavior, 19,* 105–112.

Brush, J. A., & Calkin, M. P. (2008, June 17). *Environmental interventions and dementia: Enhancing mealtimes in group dining rooms.* Retrieved from http://www.asha.org/Publication/leader/2008/080617/080617d.htm

Buchanan, R. J., Radin, D., & Huang, C. (2011). Caregiver burden among informal caregivers assisting people with multiple sclerosis. *International Journal of MS Care, 13,* 76–83. doi:10.7224/1537-2073-13.2.76

Calabresi, P. (2007). Multiple sclerosis and demyelinating conditions of the central nervous system. In L. Goldman, & D. Ausiello (Eds.), *Cecil medicine (*23rd ed, Chapter 436). Philadelphia, PA: Saunders Elsevier.

Carod-Artal, F. J., Ferreira, C. L., Trizotto, D. S., & Menezes, M. C. (2009). Burden and perceived health status among caregivers of stroke patients. *Cerebrovascular Disorders, 28,* 472–480. doi:10.1159/000 236525

Center for AIDS Prevention Studies. (1996). *Are informal caregivers important in AIDS care?* Retrieved from http://caps.ucsf.edu/resources/factsheets#Family

Center for Substance Abuse Treatment. (1998). *Substance abuse among older adults: An invisible epidemic.* Rockville, MD: Substance Abuse and Mental Health Services Administration. Treatment Improvement Protocol (TIP) Series, No. 26 (Chapter 1). Retrieved from http://www.ncbi.nlm.nih.gov/books/NBK64422

Centers for Disease Control and Prevention. (2013). *HIV among older Americans.* Retrieved from http://www.cdc.gov/hiv/risk/age/older americans/

Cherney, L. R., Gardner, P., Logemann, J. A., Newman, L. A., O-Neil-Pirozzi, T., Roth, C. R., & Solomon, N. P. (2010). The role of speech-language pathology and audiology in the optimal management of the service member returning from Iraq or Afghanistan with a blast-related head injury: Position of the communication sciences and disorders clinical trials research group. *Journal of Head Trauma Rehabilitation*, *25*, 219–224.

Code, C., & Herrmann, M. (2003). The relevance of emotional and psychosocial factors in aphasia to rehabilitation. *Neuropsychological Rehabilitation*, *13*, 109–132. doi:10.1080/09602010244000291

Cole, J. W., Pinto, A. N., Hebel, J. R., Buchholz, D. W., Earley, C. J., Johnson, C. J., . . . Kittner, S. J. (2004). Acquired immunodeficiency syndrome and the risk of stroke. *Stroke*, *35*, 51–56.

Cooke, P. (2008, June). What speech-language pathologists and caregivers can do to encourage the eating process. *SIG 13 Perspectives on Swallowing and Swallowing Disorders (Dysphagia)*, *17*, 67–73. doi:10.1044/sasd17.2.67

Cummings, J. L. (1992). Depression and Parkinson's disease: A review. *American Journal of Psychiatry*, *149*, 443–454.

Davis, F. G., Kupelian, V., Freels, S., McCarthy, B., & Surawicz, T. (2001). Prevalence estimates for primary brain tumors in the United States by behavior and major histology groups. *Neuro-Oncology*, *3*, 152–158.

Duffy, J. R. (2013). *Motor speech disorders: Substrates, differential diagnosis and management* (3rd ed.). St. Louis, MO: Elsevier Mosby.

Edwards, B. K., Howe, H. L., Ries, L. A., Thun, M. J., Rosenberg, H. M., & Feigal, E. G. (2002). Annual report to the nation on the status of cancer, 1973–1999, featuring implications of age and aging on U.S. cancer burden. *Cancer*, *94*, 2766–2792.

Ellis, C., Dismuke, C., & Edwards, K. (2010). Longitudinal trends in aphasia in the United States. *Neurorehabilitation*, *27*, 327–333. doi:10.3233/NRE-20100616

Epilepsy Foundation. (2014). *Refractory epilepsy*. Retrieved from http://www.epilepsy.com/learn/refractory-epilepsy

Family Caregivers Alliance National Center on Caregiving. (2001). *Incidence and prevalence of the major causes of brain impairment*. Retrieved from https://www.caregiver.org/incidence-and-prevalence-major-causes-brain-impairment

Figved, N., Myhr, K. M., Larsen, J. P., & Aarsland, D. (2007). Caregiver burden in multiple sclerosis: The impact of neuropsychiatric symptoms. *Journal of Neurology, Neurosurgery, & Psychiatry*, *78*, 1097–1102.

Fink, R. B., Brecher, A., Sobel, P., & Schwartz M. F. (2005) Computer-assisted treatment of word retrieval deficits in aphasia. *Aphasiology*, *19*, 943–954.

Freed, D. (2012). *Motor speech disorders: Diagnosis and treatment* (2nd ed.). Clifton Park, NY: Delmar.

Galvin, J. E., Duda, J. E., Kaufer, D. I., Lippa, C. F., Taylor, A., & Zarit, S. H. (2010). Lewy body dementia: Caregiver burden and unmet needs. *Alzheimer Disease and Associated Disorders, 24*, 177–181. doi:10.1097/WAD.0b013e3181c72b5d

Gauthier, A., Vignola, A., Calvo, A., Cavallo, E., Moglia, C., & Chio, A. (2007). A longitudinal study on quality of life and depression in ALS patient caregiver couples. *Neurology, 68*, 923–926.

Gentry, T., Wallace, J., Kvarfordt, C., & Lynch, K. (2008). Personal digital assistants as cognitive aids for individuals with severe traumatic brain injury: A community-based trial. *Brain Jury, 22*, 19–24.

Geronimo, A., Stephens, H. E., Schiff, S. J., & Simmons, Z. (2014). Acceptance of brain computer interfaces in amyotrophic lateral sclerosis. *Amyotrophic Lateral Sclerosis and Frontotemporal Degeneration, 5*, 1–7.

Hain, T. (2012). *Acoustic neuroma. American Hearing Research Foundation.* Retrieved from http://american-hearing.org/disorders/acoustic-neuroma/

Halop, J. J., & Mucke, L. (2009). Epilepsy and cognitive impairment. *Archives of Neurology, 66*, 435–440.

Harezlak, J., Buchthal, S., Taylor, M., Schifitto, G., Zhong, J., Daar, E., . . . Navia, B. (2011). Persistence of HIV-associated cognitive impairment, inflammation, and neuronal injury in era of highly active antiretroviral treatment. *AIDS, 25*, 625–633. doi:10.1097/QAD.0b013e3283427da

Hegde, M. N., & Freed, D. (2011). *Assessment of communication disorders in adults.* San Diego, CA: Plural.

Helfer, T. M., Jordan, N. N., Lee, R. B., Pietrusiak, P., Cave, K., & Schairer, K. (2011). Noise-induced hearing injury and comorbidities among postdeployment U.S. army soldiers: April 2003–2009. *American Journal of Audiology, 20*, 33–41.

Hermann, B., & Seidenberg, M. (2007) Epilepsy and cognition. *Epilepsy Currents, 7*, 1–6. Retrieved from http://www.ncbi.nlm.nih.gov/pmc/articles/PMC1797884/

Hillman, L. (2013). Caregiving in multiple sclerosis. *Physical Medicine and Rehabilitation Clinics of North America, 24*, 619–627. doi:10.1016/j.pmr.2013.06.01

Hilton, R., & Leenhouts, S. (2014). *Relatives' recommendations for their information, support and training needs: From evidence to service evaluation on the aphasia care pathway.* Retrieved from http://research.ncl.ac.uk/aphasia/audit/background.pdf

Irwin, D., Lippa, C. F., & Swearer, J. M. (2007). Cognition and amyotrophic lateral sclerosis (ALS). *American Journal of Alzheimer's Disease and Other Dementias, 22*, 300–312.

Ivanyi, B., Nollet, F., Redekop, W. K., de Haan, R., Wohlgemuht, M., & deVisser, (1999). Late onset polio sequelae: Disabilities and handicaps in a population-based cohort of the 1956 poliomyelitis outbreak in the Netherlands. *Archives of Physical Medicine and Rehabilitation, 80,* 687–690.

Johnson, R. K., Hough, M. S., King, K. A., Vos, P., & Jeffs, T. (2008). Functional communication in individuals with chronic severe aphasia using augmentative communication. *Augmentative and Alternative Communication, 24,* 269–280. doi:10.1080/07434610802463957

Jönsson, A. C., Lindgren, I., Hallström, B., Norrving, B., & Lindgren, A. (2005). Determinants of quality of life in stroke survivors and their informal caregivers. *Stroke, 36,* 803–808.

Jubelt, B. (2004). Post-polio syndrome. *Current Treatment Options in Neurology, 6,* 87–93.

Jullamate, P., de Azeredo, Z., Rosenberg, E., Pául, C., & Subgranon, R. (2007). Informal stroke rehabilitation: What are the main reasons of Thai caregivers? *International Journal of Rehabilitation Research, 30,* 315–320.

Karakis, J., Cole, A. J., Montouris, G. D., Luciana, M. S., Kimford, J. M., & Piperidou, C. (2014). Caregiver burden in epilepsy: Determinants and impact. *Epilepsy Research and Treatment, 2014,* Article ID 808421. Retrieved from http://dx.doi.org/10.1155/2014/808421

Kelly-Hayes, M., Beiser, A., Kase, C. S., Scaramucci, A., D'Agostino, R. B., & Wolf, P. A. (2003). The influence of gender and age on disability following ischemic stroke: The Framingham study. *Journal of Stroke and Cerebrovascular Diseases, 12,* 119–126.

Koul, R., Corwin, M., & Hayes, S. (2005). Production of graphic symbol sentences by individuals with aphasia: Efficacy of a computer-based augmentative and alternative communication interaction. *Brain and Language, 92,* 58–77.

LaPointe, L., Murdoch, B. E., & Stierwalt, J. A. G. (2010). *Brain-based communication disorders* (pp. 81–100). San Diego, CA: Plural.

Lin, I. F., & Hsueh-Sheng, W. (2014). Patterns of coping among family caregivers of frail older adults. *Research on Aging, 36,* 603–624.

Lofwall, M. R., Schuster, A., & Strain, E. C. (2008). Changing profile of abused substances by older persons entering treatment. *Journal of Nervous and Mental Disease, 196,* 898–905. doi:10.1016/j.jsat.2006.12.018

Lublin, F. D., & Reingold, S. C. (1996). Defining the clinical course of multiple sclerosis: results of an international survey. National Multiple Sclerosis Society (USA) Advisory Committee on Clinical Trials of New Agents in Multiple Sclerosis. *Neurology, 46,* 907–911.

Manders, E., Mariën, A., & Janssen, V. (2011). Informing and supporting partners and children of persons with aphasia: A comparison of supply and demand. *Logopedics, Phoniatrics, Vocology, 36,* 139–144. doi:10.3109/14015439.2011.562534

Marsh, N. V., Kersel, D. A., Havill, J. A., & Sleigh, J. W. (2002). Caregiver burden during the year following severe traumatic brain injury. *Journal of Clinical and Experimental Neuropsychology, 24,* 434–447.

McArthur, J. C., Hoover, D. R., Bacellar, H., Miller, E. N., Cohen, B. A., & Saab, A. (1993). Dementia in AIDS patients: Incidence and risk factors. *Neurology, 43,* 2245–2252.

McNeilly, L. (2010). Communication disorders in adults with HIV/AIDS. In D. W. Swanepoel & B. Louw (Eds.), *HIV/AIDS. Related communication hearing and swallowing disorders* (pp. 173–194). San Diego, CA: Plural.

Mizusawa, H., Hirano, A., Llena, J. F., & Shintaku, M. (1988). Cerebrovascular lesions in acquired immune deficiency syndrome (AIDS). *Acta Neuropathologica, 76,* 451–457.

Montero-Odasso, M. (2006). Dysphonia as first symptom of late-onset myasthenia gravis. *Journal of General Internal Medicine, 21,* C4–C6.

Morley, D., Dummett, S., Peters, M., Kelly, L., Hewitson, P., & Jenkinson, C. (2012). Factors influencing quality of life in caregivers of people with Parkinson's disease and implications for clinical guidelines. *Parkinson's Disease,* Article ID 190901. doi:10.1155/2012/190901

Murray, L. L., & Clark, H. M. (2015). *Neurogenic disorders of language and cognition: Evidence-based clinical practice* (2nd ed.). Austin, TX: Pro-Ed.

National Institute of Alcoholism and Alcohol Abuse. (2012). *Other substance abuse.* Retrieved from http://www.niaaa.nih.gov/alcohol-health/specialpopulations-co-occurringdisorders/other-substance-abuse

National Institute of Neurological Disorders and Stroke (NINDS). (2012). *Frontotemporal dementia information page.* Retrieved from http://www.ninds.nih.gov/disorders/picks/picks.htm

National Institute of Neurological Disorders and Stroke (NINDS). (2014). *Myasthenia gravis fact sheet.* Retrieved from http://www.ninds.nih.gov/disorders/myasthenia_gravis/detail_myasthenia_avis.htm#268403153

National Multiple Sclerosis Society. (2008). *What is multiple sclerosis?* Retrieved from http://www.nationalmssociety.org/about-multiple-sclerosis/what-isms/index.aspx

Okie, S. (2005). Traumatic brain injury in the war zone. *New England Journal Medicine, 352,* 2043–2047.

Papathanasiou, I., Coppens, P., & Potagas, C. (Eds.) (2013). *Aphasia and related neurogenic communication disorders.* Sudbury, MA: Jones and Bartlett.

Payne, J. C. (2014). *Adult neurogenic language disorders. Assessment and treatment. A comprehensive ethnobiological approach* (2nd ed., pp. 93–174). San Diego, CA: Plural.

Payne, J. C., Wright-Harp, W., & Davis, A. (2014). Traumatic brain injury. In J. C. Payne (Ed.), *Adult neurogenic language disorders. Assessment and treatment. A comprehensive, ethnobiological approach* (2nd ed., pp. 175–264). San Diego, CA: Plural.

Perry, B. P., Gantz, B. J., & Rubinstein, J. T. (2001). Acoustic neuromas in the elderly. *Otology and Neurotology, 22,* 389–391.

Prater, C. D., & Zylstra, R. G. (2006). Medical care of adults with mental retardation. *American Family Physician, 73,* 2175–2183.

Rabkin, J. G., Albert, S. M., Rowland, L. P., & Mitsumoto, H. (2009). How common is depression among ALS caregivers: A longitudinal study. *Amyotrophic Lateral Sclerosis, 10,* 448–455. doi:10.1080/1748 2960802459889.

Radunovic, A., Annane, D., Jewitt, K., & Musfa, N. (2009). Mechanical ventilation for amyotrophic lateral sclerosis/motor neuron disease. *Cochrane Database of Systematic Reviews* 2009, Issue 4. Art. No.: CD004427. doi:10.1002/14651858.CD004427.pub2

Ramasubbu, R., Robinson, R. G., Flint, A. J., Kosier, T., & Price, T. R. (1998). Functional impairment associated with acute poststroke depression: The Stroke Data Bank Study. *Journal of Neuropsychiatry and Clinical Neurosciences, 10,* 26–33.

Remy, P., Doder, M., Lees, A., Turjanski, N., & Brooks, D. (2005). Depression in Parkinson's disease: Loss of dopamine and noradrenaline innervation in the limbic system. *Brain, 128,* 1314–1322.

Riedijk, S. R., De Vugt, M. E., Duivnvoorden, H. J., Niermeijer, M. F., Van Swieten, J. C., & Tibben, A. (2006). Caregiver burden, health-related quality of life and coping in dementia caregivers: A comparison of frontotemporal dementia and Alzheimer's disease. *Dementia and Geriatric Cognitive Disorders, 22,* 405–412. doi:10.1159/000095750

Ripich, D. N., & Horner, J. (2004, April). The neurodegenerative dementias: Diagnoses and interventions. *The ASHA Leader.*

Romo González, R. J., Chaves, E., & Copello, H. (2010). Dysphagia as the sole manifestation of myasthenia gravis. *Acta Gastroenterologica Latinoamerica, 40,* 156–158.

Ross, S., & Morris, R. G. (1988). Psychological adjustment of the spouses of aphasic stroke patients. *International Journal of Rehabilitation Research, 11,* 383–386.

Rowland, L. P., & Shneider, N. E. (2001). Amyotrophic lateral sclerosis. *New England Journal of Medicine, 344,* 1688–1700. doi:10.1056/NEJM200105313442207

Schrag, A., Hovris, A., Morley, D., Quinn, N., & Jahanshahi, M. (2006). Caregiver burden in Parkinson's disease is closely associated with psychiatric symptoms, falls, and disability. *Parkinsonism & Related Disorders, 12,* 35–41.

Schubart, J. R., Kinzie, M. A., & Farace, E. (2008). Caring for the brain tumor patient: Family caregiver burden and unmet needs. *Neuro-Oncology, 11*, 61–72.

Segal, M. E., & Schall, R. R. (1996). Life satisfaction and caregiving stress for individuals with stroke and their primary caregivers. *Rehabilitation Psychology, 41*, 303–320. doi:10.1037/0090-5550.41.4.303

Shafi, N., & Carozza, L. (2012, July). Treating cancer-related aphasia. *The ASHA Leader.*

Shekim, L. (1990). Dementia. In L. L. LaPointe (Ed.), *Aphasia and related neurogenic language disorders* (pp. 210–220). New York, NY: Thieme Medical.

Small, J. A., Gutman, G., Makela, S., & Hillhouse, B. (2003). Effectiveness of communication strategies used by caregivers of persons with Alzheimer's disease during activities of daily living. *Journal of Speech, Language, and Hearing Research, 46*, 353–367. doi:10.1044/1092-4388(2003/028)

Sobel, B. P. (2001). Bingo vs. physical intervention in stimulating short-term cognition in Alzheimer's disease patients. *American Journal of Alzheimer's Disease and Other Dementias, 16*, 115–120.

Strutt, A. M., Palcic, J., Wager, J. G., Titus, C., Macadam, C., & York, M. K. (2012). Cognition, behavior, and respiratory function in amyotrophic lateral sclerosis. *ISRN Neurology, 912123*. doi:10.5402/2012/912123

Substance Abuse and Mental Health Services Administration. (2013). *Results from the 2012 National Survey on Drug Use and Health: Summary of national findings*, NSDUH Series H-46, HHS Publication No. (SMA) 13-4795. Rockville, MD: Author. Retrieved from http://www.samhsa.gov/data/NSDUH/2012SummNatFindDetTables/NationalFindings/NSDUHresults2012.htm#fig8.6

Swanepoel, D. W., & Louw, B. (2010). *HIV/AIDS related communication, hearing, and swallowing disorders.* San Diego, CA: Plural.

Tanner, D. C. (2008). *Case studies in dysphagia malpractice litigation.* San Diego, CA: Plural.

Tárraga, L., Boada, M., Modinos, G., Espinosa, A., Diego, S., Morera, A., & Becker, J. T. (2006). A randomised pilot study to assess the efficacy of an interactive, multimedia tool of cognitive stimulation in Alzheimer's disease. *Journal of Neurology, Neurosurgery, and Psychiatry, 77*, 1116–1121.

Turner, H. A., & Catania, J. A. (1997) Informal caregiving to persons with AIDS in the United States: Caregiver burden among central cities residents eighteen to forty-nine years old. *American Journal of Community Psychology, 25*, 35–59.

Vetter, P. H., Krauss, S., Steiner, O., Kropp, P., Möller, W. D., Moises, H. W., & Köller, O. (1999).Vascular dementia versus dementia of

Alzheimer's type: Do they have differential effects on caregivers' burden? *Journals of Gerontology: Series B, 54B,* S93–S98. doi:10.1093/geronb/54B.2.S93

Vincent, A., & Newsom-Davis, J. (2007). Disorders of neuromuscular transmission. In L. Goldman & D. Ausiello (Eds.), *Cecil medicine* (23rd ed., Chap. 448). Philadelphia, PA: Saunders Elsevier.

Wallace, G. L. (1993). Adult neurogenic disorders. In D. E. Battle (Ed.), *Communication disorders in multicultural populations* (pp. 239–255). Boston, MA: Andover Medical.

Wallace, G. L. (2006, July 11). Blast injury basics: A primer for the medical speech-language pathologist. *The ASHA Leader.*

Wertz, R. T., & Katz, R. C. (2004). Outcomes of computer provided treatment for aphasia. *Aphasiology, 18,* 229–244.

Wheless, J. W. (2006). Intractable epilepsy: A survey of patients and caregivers. *Epilepsy & Behavior, 8,* 756–764.

Williams, D. (2014). Maximizing outcomes in a group treatment of aphasia. *Perspectives on Neurophysiology and Neurogenic Speech and Language Disorders, 24,* 100–105.

Williamson, G. M., & Schulz, R. (1993). Coping with specific stressors in Alzheimer's disease caregiving. *Gerontologist, 33,* 747–755. doi:10.1093/geront/33.6.747

Wilson, R., Rochon, E., Milhailidis, A., & Leonard, C. (2012). Examining success of communication strategies used by formal caregivers assisting individuals with Alzheimer's disease during an activity of daily living. *Journal of Speech, Language, and Hearing Research, 55,* 328–341. doi:10.1044/10924388(2011/10-0206)

Wooten-Bielski, K. (1999). HIV and AIDS in older adults. *Geriatric Nursing, 20,* 268–272.

Wright Willis, A., Evanoff, B. A., Lian, M., Criswell, S. R., & Racette, B. A. (2010). Geographic and ethnic variation in Parkinson disease: A population-based study of US Medicare beneficiaries. *Neuroepidemiology, 34,* 143–151. doi: 10.1159/000275491

Yasuda, K., Kuwabara, K., Kuwahara, N., Abe, S., & Tetsutani, N. (2009) Effectiveness of personalized reminiscence photo videos for individuals with dementia. *Neuropsychological Rehabilitation, 19,* 603–619.

5

What Audiologists Should Know

Jay R. Lucker, Ronald C. Pearlman, and Joan C. Payne

Hearing loss is one of the most common maladies of adults, particularly as they age. According to the National Institute on Deafness and Other Communication Disorders (NIDCD, 2010a), the following are true:

- Men are more likely to experience hearing loss than women.
- Of adults ages 65 and older in the United States, 12.3% of men and nearly 14% of women are affected by tinnitus. Tinnitus is identified more frequently in non-Hispanic white individuals, and the prevalence of tinnitus is almost twice as frequent in the South as in the Northeast.
- Approximately 17% (36 million) of American adults report some degree of hearing loss.
- There is a strong relationship between age and reported hearing loss: 18% of American adults 45 to

64 years old, 30% of adults 65 to 74 years old, and 47% of adults 75 years old or older have a hearing loss.

• Only one out of five people who could benefit from a hearing aid actually wears one.

The NIDCD (2010a) estimates that approximately 15% (26 million) of Americans between the ages of 20 and 69 have a high-frequency hearing loss caused by exposure to loud sounds or noise at work or in leisure activities. Approximately 95% of those living in residential care facilities have a hearing loss that interferes with communication (Hull, 2001; Price & Gooberman-Hill, 2012).

Often, caregivers view aging adults with hearing impairments in their care in an unfavorable way, what Wallhagen calls the stigma of hearing loss (2010). In her view, this stigma causes denial of the hearing impairment and a reluctance to seek treatment or to comply with recommendations for treatment, such as wearing hearing aids. However, great individual differences are actually abundant within groups of hearing impaired adults. The caregiver needs to become aware of the types of hearing loss, the value of support before and after an audiological evaluation, and the negative consequences of stigmatizing the individual with a hearing loss.

Research has shown that a hearing loss can decrease the quality of life in older adults (Mulrow et al., 1990). In an earlier study, Wolfhart Niemeyer (1973) developed a model of psychological aspects of deteriorated hearing which shows the speaker's perception and the processing of the hearing impaired listener (Figure 5–1). This dynamic often takes place when normal hearing persons communicate with a hearing impaired individual. According to Niemeyer (1973), when a normal hearing person attempts to interact with an individual with limited or no hearing, the hearing impaired person may be perceived to have limited intelligence, or to be "dumb." This pejorative perception is internalized, causing more social isolation and misunderstanding. Eventually, both parties communicate less, and effective interpersonal communication is lost. Caregivers should be made aware of this interaction.

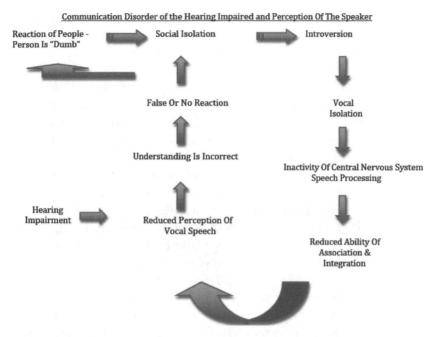

Figure 5–1. Niemeyer's model of psychological aspects of deteriorated hearing. Reprinted with permission from Maico Diagnostics.

Hearing Loss and Aging

Hearing plays a vital role in communication between the caregiver and a person receiving care. Hearing loss eventually affects how people who are elderly are able to communicate successfully with others, including their caregivers. Yet, hearing loss is only a part of the deterioration that older adults may have related to understanding what they hear, especially when they have chronic illnesses and disabilities.

Hearing loss in adults may stem from a variety of age-related changes in the peripheral and central auditory systems as well as from cognitive changes (Humes, 2008). Data from studies of older adults suggest that hearing loss may be prevalent in 25% to 30% of persons aged 65 to 74 (Bess, Lichtenstein, & Logan, 1991); yet, it may be as high as 45.9% of the population of persons aged 65 and over (Cruickshanks et al., 1998; Dalton et al., 2003). It is anticipated that as the aging population increases and as more adults live to older ages, the incidence and prevalence of hearing loss will increase as well. Known correlates for prevalence of hearing impairment are noise exposure, diabetes, and a history of strokes, among other factors (Frisina, Mapes, Kim, Frisina, & Frisina, 2006). Additionally, normal age-related changes can lead to decreases in hearing, particularly changes in the 8th cranial nerve pathways, changes in the middle ossicles, and reduction of inner ear cilia and endolymph.

There may be ethnic differences in the prevalence of hearing loss. Investigators found hearing loss greater than 25 dB in the better ear in two thirds of adults. According to Lin and others (2011), non-Hispanic whites have significantly high incidences of hearing loss and severe bilateral hearing impairment. In comparison, African Americans are less likely to have hearing loss, even mild hearing losses. This discrepancy in hearing loss prevalence between these two groups may be due to protective components in melanin (Lin, Thorpe, Gordon-Salant, & Ferruci, 2011) and has been corroborated by the National Health Interview Data results (Lee et al., 2007).

Central Hearing Loss or Auditory Processing Deficits in the Elderly

Not only does peripheral hearing decrease with aging, but age-related changes in the structures of the brain may affect how speech may be processed. These age-related changes reflect a typical deterioration in neural functioning (Mendelson & Ricketts, 2001; Pichora-Fuller, 2003; Popelar, Groh, Pelanova, Canlon, & Syka, 2006). For example, a person may have a mild, high-frequency sensorineural hearing loss, but with changes in neural structures and connections within the brain, incoming speech may be distorted further and become difficult to comprehend. Hearing aids, which merely amplify components of the incoming signal, will not clarify this distortion because the person may hear everything that is said but may not understand what is being spoken. This would be comparable to turning on an analog radio with the station slightly out of tune. An individual can certainly hear someone speaking but may not be able to decipher the spoken words.

Another central deficit that may occur for people who age is a loss in processing speed (Pichora-Fuller, 2003). Processing speed has to do with how rapidly the central nervous system is able to handle the amount of information presented. An example is when someone becomes excited and tells five different things that have just occurred that caused the excitement. The person may be speaking rapidly, too rapidly for even a normal hearing person to catch everything that was said. However, if the central auditory processing mechanisms are able to handle the speed and load (i.e., amount of information presented), it is possible for an adult with normal language, auditory processing, and cognitive abilities to understand most of what is being said and to get the general message.

This processing speed becomes more difficult for older adults, particularly those with neurological disabilities. With brain damage, the central auditory system does not work as fast as the normal system, and it is likely that language and cognitive functioning are also compromised. Hence, the listener may hear an excited person speaking and may also realize that the conversation is about different events that occurred. However, cognitive deficits and auditory processing disorders may cause the listener to experience overload and simply detach from the conversation.

Auditory processing disorders (APDs) may exist in the absence of hearing loss for older adults. That is, a person may have age-appropriate hearing (only a slight deterioration in peripheral auditory functioning) but advanced deterioration of central auditory functioning. The effect is that person is suspected of having a hearing loss. More importantly, the individual has greater difficulties in interpreting what is heard because verbal messages are significantly distorted. The difference is that age cohorts with impaired hearing without APDs are able to compensate better for any distortions that may occur due to their hearing loss.

For many older adults, aging in the absence of significant hearing loss has little effect on speech perception. However, impairment in the central auditory system can alter auditory signal processing and contribute to difficulties in understanding and processing verbal language (Garstecki & Erler, 1999; Musiek

& Chermak, 2007). When considering central auditory processes, it is important for caregivers to realize that hearing is not the only facility that is involved in comprehension. Memory and attention play important roles in comprehension as well.

As one listens, the individual has to remember what is heard and, eventually, to integrate the pieces of verbal information heard to form the unified whole for comprehension (Lucker 2010, 2011a, 2011b). There is a documented relationship between memory and hearing loss (Barzagan & Barbie, 1994). Hence, the better the memory, the better is the understanding of what we hear, and vice versa.

Not only is memory a cognitive process that affects our processing of verbal information, attention is also important. Attention and memory may decline with age (Trembley & Ross, 2007) and coexist with hearing loss. Responses from an older adult may reflect both attention deficits and hearing loss, leading to many frustrations between caregivers and care recipients (Wallhagen, Strawbridge, Shema, & Kaplan, 2004). The results can be catastrophic.

Relationship Between Hearing, Cognition, and Functioning in the Elderly

Hearing loss can mimic dementia in older adults and interfere with successful functional recovery. Central auditory dysfunction has been shown to precede dementia in a significant number of cases which suggests that this disorder may be an early marker for dementia (Gates, Cobb, Linn, Rees, Wolf, & D'Agostino, 1996; Lin, Metter, O'Brien, Resnick, Zendermen, & Ferrucci, 2011).

Hearing loss can also erode independence in functional skills. The interplay between cognition, hearing, and functional independence was investigated by Grisso, Schwarz, Wolfson, Polansky, and La Pann (1992) who found that hearing loss in older adults was a major predictor of poor physical recovery after hospitalization and contributed greatly to functional limitations. Hearing loss is also categorized as a reversible dementia because adults with significant auditory loss may show depression, disorientation, difficulty with new learning, and increased speech irrelevance (Tonkovich, 1988), especially when the central deterioration adds to comprehension difficulties.

Hearing loss may be a predictor of other cognitive disorders as adults age and may differentiate cognitive abilities between men and women. Agrawal, Platz, and Niparko (2008) observed that as men and women age, the prevalence of high-frequency sensorineural hearing loss also increases. Lin, Thorpe, Gordon-Salant, and Ferrucci (2011) reported a reduction in cognitive performance among subjects 60 to 69 years of age which was associated with a greater than 25-dB hearing loss. When cognitive decline was assessed using a standardized neuropsychological test, subjects with hearing loss performed significantly poorer than their normal hearing age cohorts. This finding suggests that hearing loss may be a significant risk factor in older adults or even an early marker of cognitive loss, likely because of age-related deterioration in central auditory functioning and APD.

Impact of Auditory Problems on Aging Adults

Older adults with hearing loss rate themselves poorly in both mental and physical health. This was particularly true for adults with bilateral loss in the Blue Mountain study. Those with hearing loss who completed the *Short Form Health Survey* revealed lower scores in both physical and mental domains compared with their normal hearing cohorts (Chia, Wang, Rochtchina, & Cumming, 2007).

Sensory impairments, such as unaided hearing loss, prevent adults from being independent and can make them vulnerable to falls and problems with equilibrium (Rubenstein, 2006). As many Americans age, declines in reaction time, diminution of visual acuity and depth perception, reduced speed of processing, and other age-related health problems can be complicated by loss of hearing. The clinical picture is worsened by the possible effects of neurological pathologies.

Impact of Auditory Problems on Caregivers

Hearing loss can create serious interpersonal communication problems that affect both the patient and those providing care. Verbal interactions between caregivers and persons in their care who have compromised auditory functioning (i.e., hearing loss and APD) are often a source of communication breakdown.

As an example, Morgan-Jones (2001) explored the effects of hearing loss in 11 married couples and five single or divorced individuals. Her findings confirm that hearing loss has the potential to disrupt intimate relationships. Several of the single/divorced subjects blamed hearing loss for the breakup of their marriages while one couple divorced shortly after the study ended.

Hence, hearing loss is only a part of what interferes with successful communication in adults, especially those with chronic illnesses and disabilities. APD can interfere and may be the most disruptive influence on interpersonal communication. Family caregivers of older persons who see audiologists for hearing testing and the fitting and adjustment of hearing aids will need to understand the impact of hearing loss and APD on communication.

What Audiologists Need to Do

Lucker and Molloy (2009) surveyed families who were caregivers to children, adolescents, and adults with XY chromosome variations. Although the care recipients were not older adults, the outcomes from this survey are important to understanding the frustrations that caregivers often feel when trying to obtain help for the people for whom they are providing care. The survey used in the study asked caregivers to identify sources of appropriate information about caring for their children. Additionally, the survey asked about the type of information provided, and requested that subjects rank-order the level of appropriateness of the type of information provided. Sources of information included medical personnel, allied health professionals (which included audiologists), psychologists, counselors, and educators (i.e., teachers, school personnel).

It was not surprising that medical professionals were identified as providing the greatest amount of medical information, but the rating was only just above the middle (helpful rather than very helpful). When ranking all four professional groups, allied health professionals were ranked equally low with medical professionals and psychologists. Counselors ranked first as the professionals from whom the most helpful information was obtained by the caregivers. Educators ranked second, but this may have been the result of responses by parents whose adult children were graduating from or no longer in the school setting. What this survey indicated was that caregivers—that is, family members who provide daily care for people with multiple disabilities including APD problems and communication deficits—need information, want information, and feel that they are not receiving appropriate information from primary or allied health professionals.

The most helpful assistance came from counselors and educators. However, the data showed that these professionals were not judged to be at the highest levels of helpfulness. The areas of concern were providing information about the medical problems involved, relating the learning, and thus, cognitive problems involved, and, most importantly, determining the communication difficulties involved when dealing with the people to whom they provide care.

Caregivers may not feel they are obtaining helpful information, especially from audiologists and other allied health professionals. Therefore, audiologists need to learn about the needs of caregivers and not merely focus on the needs of their clients. It is not enough to reprogram a hearing aid when a caregiver complains about problems communicating effectively with the person who is using the hearing aid. Caregivers need help in understanding the reasons for the breakdown in communication between themselves and the persons to whom they are providing care. They need to understand methods to be effective and appropriate in communicating with these elderly persons. But, they also need someone who cares about them and their feelings, frustrations, and needs. Various chapters in this book can help audiologists better understand how to work successfully with caregivers and not merely focus on the person with the hearing problem.

Hearing and Balance Disorders

Hearing and balance disorders are particularly stressful for caregivers because in addition to a possible hearing loss, loss of balance can result in falls that can cause traumatic brain injuries

(TBIs) or fractures of hips and limbs. Home safety measures can decrease the possibility of falls in the home.

The vestibular labyrinth of the inner ear functions to detect tilts of the head and head rotation (Bear, Connors & Paradiso, 2006). Sudden-onset vertigo can occur as a result of lesion sites in the circulatory system to the posterior portion of the brain, specifically, the vertebral and basilar arteries and their branches (Shepherd, 2007). Also, as adults age, the vestibular system in the inner ear (which interacts with the muscles of eye movement and the cerebellum to detect linear and angular acceleration of the head as in standing and walking) begins to lose nerve cells from about age 55. Blood flow to the vestibular system also decreases with age. The gradual, age-related loss of vestibular nerve endings can result in severe balance problems without any associated dizziness or vertigo. This type of slow loss of vestibular function may be first noticed as difficulty walking or standing, especially in the dark while on soft or uneven surfaces, such as a thick carpet or a forest path (Vestibular Disorders Association, n.d.).

Of all of the vestibular disorders, benign paroxysmal positional vertigo (BPPV) is one of the most common in older adults. BPPV is due to displacement of otolithic crystals into the posterior semicircular canal in the inner ear. With head movement, the displaced otolithic crystals shift, sending false signals to the brain that lead to dizziness or vertigo (Seiden, Tami, Penssak, Cotton & Gluckman, 2000. Symptoms of BPPV are almost always precipitated by a change in head position. Getting out of bed and rolling over in bed are two common problem motions that trigger vertigo and nystagmus (involuntary eye movements). Some people feel dizzy and unsteady when they tip their heads back to look up (Fife et al., 2008; Ko, Hoffman, & Sklare, 2006).

Ménière's disease is another inner ear disorder involving the vestibular system that causes vertigo, tinnitus, a feeling of fullness, and sensorineural hearing loss that lasts for more than 24 hours. The disease usually affects only one ear (NIDCD, 2010b). Ménière's disease produces a recurring set of symptoms as a result of abnormally large amounts of a fluid, endolymph, collecting in the inner ear. The tinnitus is typically described as a roaring sound that becomes louder prior to the onset of vertigo.

Hearing loss typically follows the configuration of low-frequency sensorineural hearing loss which commonly fluctuates. Many patients describe a sensation of aural fullness or pressure prior to the onset of vertigo, which may be accompanied by tinnitus. Episodes of vertigo typically last at least 20 minutes and may persist for up to several hours.

The incidence of Ménière's disease (number of new cases per year) is difficult to assess. Estimates vary widely, in part because of the variability in diagnostic criteria across studies. The prevalence, however (all cases within a population), is generally known to increase with age (NIDCD, 2010b).

Other vestibular disorders that may occur in older adults include vestibular neuritis (inflammation of the vestibular branch of the vestibulo-cochlear nerve, resulting in dizziness or vertigo but no change in hearing) and ototoxicity (exposure to certain chemicals that damage the inner ear or the vestibulo-cochlear nerve, which sends balance and hearing information from the inner ear to the brain). Ototoxicity can result in temporary or permanent disturbances of hearing, balance, or both (Cone et al., n.d.).

Summary

Hearing loss and APD can severely compromise the independence of adults, particularly older adults, in the areas of daily functioning and interpersonal communication. These disabilities can also affect how well caregivers can assist an adult with a hearing impairment when there has been a communication breakdown. Such problems are exacerbated when the auditory problems coexist with other health problems and with cognitive and other related brain changes that accompany aging.

Both hearing loss and APD can mimic dementia or may be early signs of impending dementia. Older adults often do not wear their hearing aids and have little understanding about APD problems. There is a need, therefore, for audiologists to help patients and their caregivers appreciate the value of successful auditory comprehension and better, more age-sensitive aural rehabilitation in daily communication. This means that audiologists need to focus on how to effectively listen to, deal with, and interact with caregivers and not merely focus their services on the adult client with the auditory problem.

Vertigo and Ménière's disease can complicate the quality of life for an older person and the family caregiver. Neural changes in the vestibular system and ototoxicity are known causes of problems with equilibrium and hearing loss that can result in falls and other complications from associated head, limb, and hip injuries. For these persons, family caregivers will need information on home safety measures, for example, removing loose rugs and increasing lighting on stairs and in hallways, to decrease the likelihood of falls.

Assisting Caregivers to Manage Hearing Amplification

When a hearing loss or auditory processing disorder is diagnosed, caregivers should schedule a hearing test every year both for baseline functioning and to detect changes in hearing functioning. A hearing test performed by an audiologist should be emphasized. Hearing loss is often an insidious process and changes in hearing acuity may go unrecognized by an older adult who feels that, "People don't speak as clearly as they did years ago." Other complications may arise such as impacted earwax (cerumen) which can cause a sudden decline in hearing when the wax softens after a shower and completely seals off the ear canal. With some training, a caregiver may find it easy to use an otoscope to view the ear canal and determine if earwax is the cause of the sudden hearing loss.

Hearing Aids

One approach to decreasing hearing loss is through amplification through hearing aids and cochlear implants. As the population ages, both devices will increase in use as both technologies continue to evolve. A hearing aid often means the difference between an active social life as opposed to reclusive isolation

(Popelka et al., 1998). Care of cochlear implants will require professional attention. However, the caregiver can often provide solutions to malfunctioning hearing aids if a few basic steps are taken to determine the cause of the malfunction. Troubleshooting a hearing aid is straightforward.

A hearing aid should be listened to by the caregiver every day to make sure it is operating properly. A hearing aid stethoscope, like the one pictured in Figure 5–2, can be attached to any hearing aid so that the caregiver can listen to the device without needing to place the hearing aid into the caregiver's ear. A hearing aid stethoscope is inexpensive and can be purchased from any company that sells hearing aid accessories.

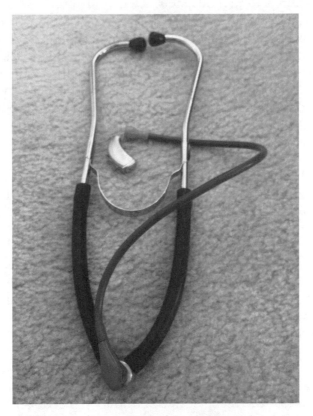

Figure 5–2. Hearing aid stethoscope used to listen to a hearing aid.

Hearing aids produced in the last several years are digital and have built-in processors that can automatically change listening programs without intervention from the user, depending on the listening situation. Separate programs can be set for church, theater, music, and restaurants, to name just a few listening environments. After a history of the patient's hearing loss is obtained, which includes information about the person's lifestyle, and a full audiometric examination is completed by the audiologist, a determination can be made for a prescription of the hearing aid that serves the best advantage of the patient.

Costs for hearing aids are not just the cost of the aid itself, but include the audiologist's professional services as well. Often the hearing aid will need adjustments and may also need repairs; these situations cannot be ameliorated with amplification devices that were purchased through the Internet or by mail order. Bargain hearing aids may not turn out to be a bargain without an audiologist who can prescribe, adjust, and service the instrument.

Hearing aids consist of four general parts: (a) a microphone that changes sound to electrical energy (there may be two microphones: directional and omnidirectional); (b) an amplifier that increases the loudness of the sound and changes the program of the hearing aid to adjust to background noise and optimum listening conditions using one of several digital settings; (c) a receiver that acts like a speaker and converts the electrical energy from the amplifier back into sound; and (d) the battery that powers the unit. In addition to the four general parts, there are user adjustment controls in some hearing aids. Hearing aids may be configured in several different ways, for example, over the ear (OTE), in the ear (ITE), or completely in the ear canal (CIC) hearing aids. The components may be in different places depending on the type of aid, but the components are, essentially, all the same. The owner's manual often has a diagram showing the major components.

An ear mold in some cases is needed to maintain the hearing aid in the ear. It may help prevent a high-pitched squealing sound called *feedback* which is caused when the microphone feeds sound to the receiver in a sound loop. Feedback indicates a poorly fitted ear mold that does not create a sound barrier to the receiver. In such a case, the audiologist should readjust the ear mold.

The caregiver should be instructed to keep spare batteries handy so a drained battery can be replaced. If rechargeable batteries are used, fully charged batteries should be readily available in the event that the battery in use is depleted. Batteries come in several sizes depending on the requirements of the hearing aid. Sizes of batteries include 10, 13, 312, and 675. Modern batteries are mercury free and produce energy by a zinc-air chemistry. Zinc-air batteries use air to mix with the zinc in order to create a charge. Zinc-air batteries come with a paper that has a sticky backing attached to the battery to prevent air from entering the battery and activating it. The paper should not be removed until just before using the battery. Batteries should fit into the hearing aid battery compartment easily. Forcing the battery into the hearing aid will likely damage the battery compartment. If the battery does not slide in easily, the battery should be turned upside down with the paper removed and then reinserted. A swallowed battery is life threatening, so it should be kept away from children and animals. If a caregiver believes that a battery was swallowed, the poison control center should be called immediately at 1-800-222-1222.

A hearing aid can be tested by cupping a hearing aid in both hands to determine if it is working (Figure 5–3). If the aid

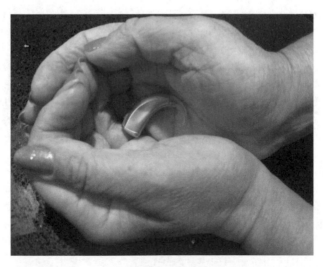

Figure 5–3. Cupping both hands to create feedback.

is amplifying sound, squealing caused by feedback should be heard. If feedback is not heard, the caregiver should replace the battery.

If the battery is still functioning but the hearing aid is not working, the caregiver should inspect the receiver. If earwax is clogged in the receiver or ear mold, the hearing aid may not function. A tool that comes with the aid may be used to clear the cerumen from the receiver or ear mold. Caregivers should be cautioned not to go too deep and damage the receiver. A light brushing away of the wax is all that may be needed to cause the aid to function again. If the receiver or ear mold is free of wax and the battery is fresh, the hearing aid should be working. In the event the aid is not working, it should be returned to the audiologist for repair.

Caregivers should be told that hearing aids should not be worn when the wearer is sleeping. New hearing aids are water resistant but not waterproof. Thus, they should not be worn during showering, morning washing, or in heavy rain. At night, the hearing aid battery compartment can be opened to prevent continued discharge of the battery. If possible, the hearing aid should be placed overnight in a closed container with desiccants, or prepackaged solids that absorb water to dry out the components. A soft cloth or tissue can be used to wipe dirt and grease from the hearing aid.

A cautionary note to caregivers: hearing aids will not permit the patient to hear as they did in their teens. Using a hearing aid cannot repair most of the damage to the biological hearing system or the auditory nerves. Hearing aids must work through a biological system that may have its own inherent distortion. Much of the background noise in a room or on the street is amplified along with the signal the patient is trying to hear when wearing a hearing aid. Having the hearing aid user conversing in a quiet area can be very helpful. Some patients may be reading lips without realizing they are doing so. Conversations in a well-lit area where the patient can see the face of the person talking is also helpful. For patients who have hearing loss in both ears, two hearing aids can help to perceive directionality of sound and provide stereo sound rather than have the entire sound signal going into the one amplified ear.

Cochlear Implants

For some adults with hearing loss, a hearing aid may not be sufficient in helping them hear. The person may, instead, be fitted with
a cochlear implant. The implant device differs from the hearing
aid. Whereas the hearing aid has an ear mold or molded part that
fits in the ear, cochlear implants have a device worn behind the
ear with one part fitting into the ear. The device that fits behind
the ear also has a short wire and round piece that attaches by an
internal magnet to a surgically implanted magnet that is usually
inserted behind the ear in the skull. The audiologist should advise
the caregiver on how to fit the external portion of the device
behind the ear and attach the magnet to the person's head.

As with the hearing aid, the cochlear implant also has a
battery compartment. The devices usually use multiple batteries that need to be checked for functioning and changed if the
batteries are not functioning. The audiologist will need to assist
the caregiver with using the diagram provided with the implant
to insert batteries and in securing a battery checker. A battery
checker can be obtained from companies that sell cochlear
implant accessories.

Helping Caregivers Select Assistive Devices

Many people with hearing loss find success in hearing and communicating using hearing aids or cochlear implants. However,
for others, such devices are not successful, but the people still
need help hearing and communicating. In these cases, there are
assistive devices that can be used in place of hearing aids or a
cochlear implant or as an addition to the use of an individual's
hearing device.

When a person with normal hearing is living with an individual with a hearing loss, that normal hearing person often
complains that the television or music system is uncomfortably
loud. The hard of hearing individual may also have problems
hearing on the telephone. Modern hearing aids can be equipped
with Bluetooth devices that can stream the sound of the television or telephone directly into the hearing aid. This allows the

normal hearing person to enjoy a comfortable listening level. The person with the hearing loss can adjust the loudness of the signal using the volume control as needed without bothering others. Bluetooth devices require a hearing aid accessory and may add cost to the hearing aid.

There are many other assistive devices that can help the individual with a hearing loss. Room lights that flash when the telephone or doorbell rings, telephones with built-in amplifiers, TTY (text) telephones that work like a printer over long distances showing the message on a screen, videophones, and computer programs such as Skype that allow for visualization of sign language, and story boards that take the place of a pencil and paper are just a few devices to make communication easier for the person with a hearing challenge.

Noise Suppression Circuits

Hearing aids and cochlear implants are fitted specifically for the person with the hearing loss. Both hearing aids and cochlear implants have microphones that pick up the sounds that are delivered to the ear of the listener as well as circuits tuned, or programmed, to the specific needs of that individual. However, regardless of the noise suppression circuits in hearing aids and cochlear implants, they still pick up all of the sound received by the microphone and deliver that sound to the person's ear. The noise suppression circuits can reduce the noise and some unwanted sound, but they cannot get rid of all distracting sounds for many older listeners.

Microphone and Personal Listening Device Systems

Young people wearing hearing aids or fit with cochlear implants must depend on their brains and central auditory processing mechanisms to aid in understanding speech when there is noise. However, one method for making this job even easier is to place the microphone as close to the mouth of the speaker as possible. There are two devices that provide this function, and both can be used by caregivers to help make communication with elderly adults more successful.

The first and more expensive device is called a personal FM system. This system includes two main components. One is a microphone/transmitter system that is worn by the speaker, such as the caregiver. The microphone is close to the speaker's mouth picking up what that person says while the transmitter relays the auditory message to a receiver worn by the listener. The receiver can be directly linked to the person's hearing aid or cochlear implant by a device called a boot, or the person with the hearing loss can wear headphones attached to a receiver box worn by that person. When the headphones and receiver box are used, the receiver includes an amplifier that allows for adjustment of the volume and can have filters built in to help reduce background noise that might be picked up by the microphone. However, since the person's mouth is so close to the microphone compared with any noise that might be picked up, the person's speech is always significantly louder than any noise that might be picked up and delivered which cannot be filtered out. Additionally, the earphones worn by the person with the hearing loss help filter out background noise since the earphones cover the person's ears.

When a listener uses an FM system with a boot for his or her hearing aid or cochlear implant, it is necessary to insure that the correct boot is used. The caregiver can contact the audiologist who fitted the hearing aid or cochlear implant and ask if that audiologist also fits FM systems for the device. That professional can then obtain the appropriate boot for the hearing aid or cochlear implant. If the audiologist does not fit FM systems, that professional can contact the hearing aid or cochlear implant manufacturer and identify what is the appropriate personal FM system and boot needed. Figures 5–4 and 5–5 present examples of personal FM systems connected with behind-the-ear (BTE) hearing aids and using earphones.

A personal listening device has a microphone attached to the device which also houses the amplifier. The earphones are then plugged into the amplifier box. When the caregiver wishes to speak with the person with hearing loss, the caregiver can take the box and speak directly into the microphone. Some adults may prefer ear buds rather than bulky headphones as their earphones. Ear buds are the type of listening earphone one might

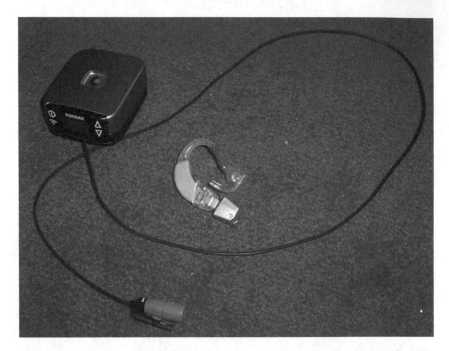

Figure 5–4. Sample personal FM system connected to hearing aid. Note the bottom part of the hearing aid which is the "boot," the "box" is the transmitter connected with the microphone. (Photo of the Phonak Campus S, Retrieved from http://www.phonak.com/com/b2c/en/products/fm.html) Permission to reprint granted.

use with an iPod. These devices do not substitute for hearing aids or cochlear implants but are available for use when the hearing aid or cochlear implant is not successfully used. Figure 5–6 presents an example of a personal listening device.

Some adults with hearing loss function successfully with their hearing aid or cochlear implant when speaking with people but have difficulties listening to TV. If the person is using an FM system, the caregiver can place the microphone of the system near the speaker on the TV. For those with hearing loss who do not use FM systems but want to enjoy TV better, there are listening devices made specifically for TV listening. These devices have special headphones attached that the listener wears. The headphones are attached to a receiver device that houses an infrared

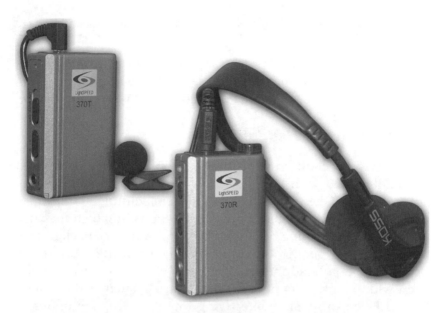

Figure 5–5. Sample personal FM system connected with earphones. The earphones are shown with the microphone/transmitter. Photo of a Lightspeed personal FM system. Reprinted with permission from Lightspeed Technologies, Inc.

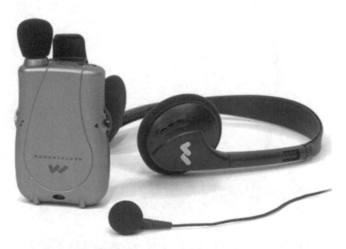

Figure 5–6. Sample personal listening device. This example can use headphones or ear buds for listening. (Photo of a William Sound Personal Listening Device, retrieved from http://www.williamsound.com/prod ucts/) Permission to reprint granted.

Red (IR) receiver. The device also uses an IR transmitter with microphone placed on the TV close to the loudspeaker of the TV. Figure 5–7 shows a sample of such an IR TV listening device.

Noise Reduction Headphones

There may be a different listening problem other than what is usually aided with hearing aids or cochlear implants. Some adults may find the use of the IR TV system helpful, but they may find that listening to music or other situations in which they use headphones disturbing because of the annoyance of background noise. For these people, the caregiver might consider purchasing noise reduction headphones. These have become very popular even with people who have normal hearing, such as those who like to listen to music while flying on airplanes. A number of

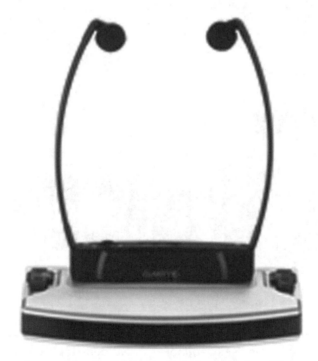

Figure 5–7. Sample IR TV listening system. (Photo of a Williams Sound system, retrieved from http://www.williamsound.com/products/) Permission to reprint granted.

companies manufacture noise reduction headphones, and the caregiver might even be able to purchase a pair through the Internet for use by a hearing impaired person. The headphones look like regular headphones, but they have a special circuit built in to reduce the annoyance of continuous background noises.

Amplified Telephones

Other persons with hearing loss may not need to use a hearing aid or cochlear implant, but have problems using the telephone. These adults cannot hear well on standard telephones, even those with volume controls and even when they put the volume to maximum. The caregiver may wish to obtain special telephones such as the following: amplified telephones that have amplification stronger than on standard phones or a videophone that provides a screen on which the person can see the speaker's face and use visual cues for speech reading to aid in understanding what that person is saying (see Figure 5–8 for sample videophone).

Visual Alerting Systems

Sometimes the problem with the phone, and even the doorbell, is not that the person with a hearing impairment cannot hear when using the phone, but the person is not able to detect that the phone is ringing or someone is at the door ringing the bell. For these adults with hearing loss, there are assistive devices that are either amplified telephones or doorbell ringers. Often, an older adult with a hearing loss will not use his or her hearing aid, cochlear implant, or personal listening system until the caretaker comes to place it in their ears. Yet, the caretaker wishes to speak with the person on the phone or stands at the door ringing the bell for a long time. Even the use of an amplified ringer is not sufficient. In such cases, there are visual alerting devices that flash lights when the telephone or doorbell rings. In such cases, a person may be alerted by such devices and then put on the hearing aid or cochlear implants to respond to the telephone or answer the door.

Many adults with a hearing loss will not sleep with the hearing aids, cochlear implants, or personal listening devices.

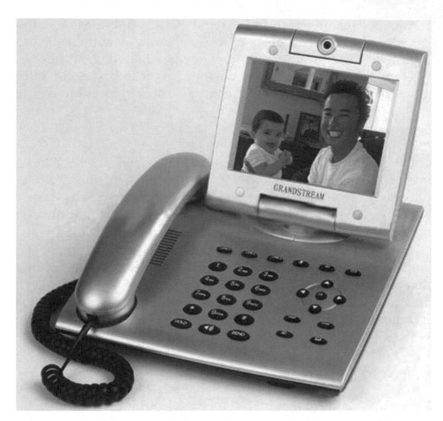

Figure 5–8. Sample videophone. (Photo of videophone retrieved from http://www.telephoneyourway.com/) Permission to reprint granted.

However, the person may want to be awake at a specific time but cannot hear the alarm clock. For such a person, the caretaker might obtain a special alarm device that uses flashing lights that flash in the darkened room to awaken the sleeper. Another device is a special bed vibrator that alerts when it is time to wake up.

There are many assistive devices that can be used along with or in place of hearing aids and cochlear implants which caregivers can use with those to whom they are providing care. There are a number of websites that caregivers and audiologists can check out that provide additional information about these assistive devices. The following is a sample of some of these websites:

- Elder Parent Help (http://www.elderparenthelp.com/guide-assistive-listening-devices): There is a very good article on this website that can be very useful, entitled "A Guide to Assistive Listening Devices/"
- Hearing Loss Association of America (HLAA) (http://www.hearingloss.org/): There is also a very good video series on assistive listening devices on their website (http://www.hearingloss.org): "Hearing Assistive Technology," which can be retrieved from http://www.hearingloss.org/content/video-series-hearing-assistive-technology
- The CLERC Center at Gallaudet University (http://www.gallaudet.edu/clerc_center/): There is very good information there on hearing aids and other assistive devices which can be retrieved from http://www.gallaudet.edu/clerc_center/information_and_resources/info_to_go/hearing_and_communication_technology/hearing_technology/hearing_aids/hearing_aids_and_other_ass_dev_where_to_get_asst.html

The various devices discussed in this section can be obtained from a variety of companies. However, the caregiver should be advised to consult with the audiologist for other resources, including the websites identified above. There are several companies that provide many of the assistive devices discussed in this section, such as Bose.

For further reading, the following article provides a comprehensive overview of assistive technology for older adults with hearing loss. The article is titled, "Candidacy and management of assistive listening devices: Special needs of the elderly," by S. A. Lessner (2003, *International Journal of Audiology, 42*[2], 68–76).

Recommendations for Talking With People With Hearing Impairments

Caregivers should be instructed that the goal when speaking with a person with a hearing loss is to maximize communication so that the listener is best able to understand what is said. The following are some suggestions for caregivers to maximize this communication:

- Have the hearing impaired person stand close to the speaker (3–5 feet) so that the speaker's voice is louder than the background noise.
- Be sure the listener can see your face and that it is well lit.
- Tell the hearing impaired person the topic of discussion if he or she is joining a conversation.
- Rephrase a sentence that is not understood; do not repeat the same sentence in the same way a second time.
- Do not speak rapidly.
- If the area in which you are conversing is noisy, direct the person with the hearing loss to a quiet area and continue the conversation.
- If there is a lot of reverberation in the room, such as in a church, have the person with the hearing loss sit in the seat closest to the speaker.
- Try to include people with hearing loss in as many social events as possible.
- If visual aids are possible, use them.
- Request that speakers use a microphone in meetings or events.
- Ask the person with the hearing loss to express his or her thoughts on a topic.
- Consider using closed captioning on the television and other media if available.
- If the listener uses sign language, have a sign language interpreter available for communication with people who do not use sign language.
- If the person with the hearing loss uses eyeglasses, be sure that person brings the glasses with them to all events.
- When conversing in a group of people, tell the others that this person has a hearing problem.
- Encourage the hearing handicapped individual to inform others of his or her hearing loss and to be

assertive in asking for help that will make the situation easier for maximizing communication.

In the end, the goal is to provide the best situations possible to maximize communication for the adult with a hearing loss. Caregivers may need to be consciously aware of all the strategies they need to use to reach this maximal situation, but in the end, it will ease the burden of those giving care.

Summary

In this chapter, information is provided for assisting caregivers with amplification and assistive devices necessary to improve communication between them and their hearing impaired care recipients. Many persons can benefit from hearing aids and cochlear implants, and caregivers should be instructed on how to manage and care for these systems. Other persons may benefit from assistive devices either alone or as a complement to amplification systems. These devices help to buffer the daily stress on caregivers with normal hearing who live with adults with hearing loss. Finally, some suggestions for communicating with persons with hearing loss are provided to assist persons with hearing loss to feel included in social interactions both with the caregiver and in group settings.

Resources

Deaf and Hard of Hearing Services (DHHS)
http://www.dhhsd.org

Telephone Equipment Distribution Program (TED)
http://www.tedprogram.org
(800) 657-3663 (VOICE)
(888) 206-6555 (TTY)

Hearing Loss Association of America (HLAA)
http://www.hearingloss.org
7910 Woodmont Avenue, Suite 1200
Bethesda, MD 20814
(301) 657-2248

American Academy of Audiology (AAA)
http://www.audiology.org
11730 Plaza America Drive, Suite 300
Reston, VA 20190
(800) 222-2336

Center for Hearing and Communication
http://www.chchearing.org
50 Broadway, 6th Floor
New York, NY 10004
(917) 305-7700 (VOICE)
(917) 305-7999 (TTY)

AARP
http://www.aarp.org
601 E. Street, NW
Washington, DC 20049
(800) 687-2277

References

Agrawal, Y., Platz, E. A., & Niparko, J. K. (2008). Prevalence of hearing loss and differences by demographic characteristics among U.S. adults. *Archives of Internal Medicine, 168*, 1522–1530.

Barbazan, M., & Barbie, A. N. (1994). The effects of depression, health, and stressful life-events on self-reported memory problems among aged blacks. *International Journal of Aging and Human Development, 38*, 351–362

Bear, M. F., Connors, B. W., & Paradiso, M. A. (2006). *Neuroscience: Exploring the brain* (3rd ed.). Philadelphia, PA: Lippincott, Williams & Wilkins.

Bess, F. H., Lichtenstein, M. J., & Logan, S. A. (1991). Audiologic assessment of the elderly. In W. Rintelmann (Ed.), *Hearing assessment* (2nd ed.). Austin, TX: Pro-Ed.

Chia, E. M, Wang, J. J., Rochtchina, E., & Cumming, R. R. (2007). Hearing impairment and health-related quality of life: The Blue Mountain Hearing Study. *Ear and Hearing, 28*, 187–195.

Cone, B., Dorn, P., Konrad-Martin, D., Lister, J., Ortiz, C., & Schairer, K. (2012). *Ototoxic medications (medication effects)*. Retrieved from http://www.asha.org/public/hearing/OtotoxicMedications/#sthash.BVa29puT.dpuf

Cruickshanks, K. J., Wiley, T. L., Tweed, T. S., Klein, B. E., Klein, R., Mares Perlman, J. A., & Nondahl, D. M. (1998). Prevalence of hearing loss in older adults in Beaver Dam, Wisconsin: The epidemiology of hearing loss study. *American Journal of Epidemiology, 148*(9), 879–886.

Dalton, D. S., Cruickshanks, K. J., Klein, B. E. K., Klein, R., Wiley, T. L., & Nondahl, D. M. (2003). The impact of hearing loss on quality of life in older adults. *Gerontologist, 43*, 661–668.

Fife, T. D., Iverson, D. J., Lempert, T., Furman, J. M., Baloh, R. W., & Gronseth, G. S. (2008). Practice parameter: Therapies for benign paroxysmal positional vertigo (an evidence-based review): Report of the Standards Subcommittee of the American Academy of Neurology. *Neurology, 70*, 2067–2074.

Frisina, S. T., Mapes, F., Kim, S. H., Frisina, D. R., & Frisina, R. D. (2006). Characterization of hearing loss in aged type II diabetics. *Hearing Research, 211*(1–2), 103–113.

Garstecki, D. C., & Erler, S. F. (1999). Older adult performance on the Communication Profile for the Hearing Impaired: Gender difference. *Journal of Speech and Hearing Research, 42*, 785–796.

Gates, G. A., Cobb, J. L., Linn, R. T., Rees, T., Wolf, P. A., & D'Agostino, R. B. (1996). Central auditory dysfunction, cognitive dysfunction, and dementia in older people. *Archives of Otolaryngology Head and Neck Surgery, 122*, 161–167.

Grisso, J. A., Schwarz, D., Wolfson, V., Polansky, M., & La Pann, K. (1992). The impact of falls in an inner-city elderly African American population. *Journal of the American Geriatric Society, 43*, 7–9.

Hull, R. H. (2001). Incidence of hearing loss in a nursing home population. Unpublished study. Wichita, KS: Wichita State University. In R. H. Hull (Ed.), *Aural rehabilitation, serving children and adults* (4th ed., pp. 426–427). San Diego, CA: Singular.

Humes. L. E. (2008, April). Aging and speech communication: Peripheral, central auditory, and cognitive factors affecting the speech-understanding problems of older adults. *The ASHA Leader.*

Ko, C., Hoffman, H. J., & Sklare, D. A. (2006). *Chronic imbalance or dizziness and falling: Results from the 1994 disability supplement to the national health interview survey and the second supplement on aging study.* Paper presented at the Annual Meeting of the Association for Research in Otolaryngology, Baltimore, MD.

Lee, D. J., Gomez-Martin, O., Lam, B. L., Zheng, D. D., Arheart, K. L., Christ, S. L., & Caban, A. J. (2007). Severity of concurrent visual and hearing impairment and mortality: The 1986–1994 National Health Interview Survey. *Journal of Aging and Health, 19*, 382–396. doi:10.1177/0898264307300174

Lin, F. R., Metter, E. J., O'Brien, R. J., Resnick, S. M., Zonderman, A. B., & Ferrucci, L. (2011). Hearing loss and incident dementia. *Archives of Neurology, 68,* 214–220.

Lin, F. R., Thorpe, R., Gordon-Salant, S., & Ferrucci, L. (2011). Hearing loss prevalence and risk factors among older adults in the United States. *The Journal of Gerontology, Series A, Biological Sciences and Medical Sciences, 66,* 582–590. doi:10.1093/gerona/glr002

Lucker, J. R. (2010). *Working with children with auditory processing disorders. Self-study course for continuing education (CEU) from the American Speech-Language-Hearing Association (ASHA), the American Psychological Association (APA), and the American Occupational Therapy Association (AOTA), Revised version.* [Available on CD through http://www.pesi.com.]

Lucker, J. R. (2011a). What are auditory processing disorders? In, H. Edell, J. R. Lucker, & L. Alderman (Eds.), *Don't you get it? Living with auditory learning disabilities.* Wood Dale, IL: Stoelting.

Lucker, J. R. (2011b). *Helping children with auditory processing disorders: Identification, management, and effective interventions. Self-study web course for continuing education (CEU) from the American Speech Language-Hearing Association (ASHA), the American Psychological Association (APA), and the American Association of Occupational Therapists (AOTA).* [Web-based course available through http://www.pesi.com.]

Lucker, J. R., & Molly, A. T. (2009). *Survey of family needs for families of children with XY chromosome variations.* Invited presentation made at the 2009 Annual Conference of Association for X and Y Chromosome Variations, Denver, CO.

Mendelson, J. R., & Ricketts, C. (2001). Age-related temporal processing speed deterioration in the auditory cortex. *Hearing Research, 158*(1–2), 84–94.

Morgan-Jones, R. (2001). *Hearing differently: The impact of hearing impairment on family life.* London, UK: Whurr.

Mulrow, C., Aguilar, C., Endicott, J., Tuley, M., Velez, R., Charlip, W., . . . DeNino, L. (1990). Quality-of-life changes and hearing impairment: A randomized trial. *Annals of Internal Medicine, 113,* 188–194.

Musiek, F. E., & Chermak, G. D. (2007). *Handbook of (central) auditory processing disorders. Vol. 1. Auditory neuroscience and diagnostics.* San Diego, CA: Plural.

National Institute on Deafness and Other Communication Disorders (NIDCD). (2010a). *Quick statistics.* Retrieved from http://www. nidcd.nih.gov/health/statistics/Pages/quick.aspx

National Institute on Deafness and Other Communication Disorders (NIDCD). (2010b). *Meniere's disease.* Retrieved from http://www.nid cd.nih.gov/health/balance/pages/meniere.aspx

Niemeyer, W. (1973). Psychological aspects of hearing-aid fitting. Part I. *Journal of Audiological Technique, 12–13*, 9–16.

Pichora-Fuller, M. K. (2003). Cognitive aging and auditory information processing. *International Journal of Audiology, 42*, 26–32.

Popelar, J., Groh, D., Pelánová, J., Canlon, B., & Syka, J. (2006). Age-related changes in cochlear and brainstem auditory functions in Fischer 344 rats. *Neurobiological Aging, 27*, 490–500.

Popelka, M. M., Cruckshanks, K. J., Wilen, T. L., Tweed, T. S., Klein, B. E., & Klein, R. (1998). Low prevalence of hearing aid use among older adults with hearing loss: The epidemiology of hearing loss study. *American Geriatric Society, 46*(9), 1075–1078.

Price, H., & Gooberman-Hill, R. (2012). "There's a hell of a noise": Living with a hearing loss in residential care. *Age and Ageing, 41*, 40–46. doi:10.1093/ageing/afr112. Epub 2011 Sep 1.

Rubenstein, L. Z. (2006). Fall in older people: Epidemiology, risk factors and strategies for prevention. *Aging and Ageing, 35*(Suppl. 2), ii37–ii41. doi:10.1093/ageing/afl084

Seiden, A. M, Tami, T. A., Penssak, M. L., Cotton, R. T., & Gluckman, J. L. (2002). *Otolaryngology, the essential text* (pp. 44–58). New York, NY: Thieme.

Shepard, N. T. (2007, May 29). Dizziness and balance disorders: The role of history and laboratory studies in diagnosis and management. *The ASHA Leader*. Retrieved from http://www.asha.org/publications/leader/2007/070529/f070529a.htm

Tonkavich, J. D. (1988). Management of communicative and swallowing disorders in nonacute settings: Home care, hospice, skilled nursing facility. In A. F. Johnson & B. H. Jacobson (Eds.), *Medical speech-language pathology: A practitioner's guide* (pp.150–175). New York, NY: Thieme.

Tremblay, K. L., & Ross, B. (2007, November). Auditory rehabilitation and the aging brain. *The ASHA Leader*.

Uhlmann, R., Larson, E., Rees, T., Koepsell, T., & Duckert, L. (1989). Relationship of hearing impairment to dementia and cognitive dysfunction in older adults. *Journal of the American Medical Association, 261*, 1916–1919.

Vestibular Disorders Association (n.d.). *Causes of dizziness.* Retrieved from http://vestibular.org/node/2

Wallhagen, M. I. (2010). The stigma of hearing loss. *Gerontologist, 50*, 66–75.

Wallhagen, M. I., Strawbridge, W. J., Sherma, S. J., & Kaplan, G. A. (2004). Impact of self-assessed hearing loss on a spouse: A longitudinal analysis. *Journal of Gerontology, 59*, 190.

Yueh, B., Shapiro, N., MacLean, C. H., & Shekelle, P. G. (2003). Screening and management of adult hearing loss in primary care. *Journal of the American Medical Association, 289*(15), 1976–1985.

6

Identifying and Assessing the Impact of Caregiving

Joan C. Payne

Initial Data Gathering

Effective and comprehensive assessment is a key step to determining appropriate support services for family caregivers, especially when the patient's plan of care depends on the contributions of family members. With the movement toward person- and family-centered care, there is growing recognition of the need to expand assessment of the individual with chronic or disabling conditions to include assessment of the family (Feinberg & Houser, 2012). Speech-language pathologists and audiologists should be knowledgeable about the types of assessments that are designed for caregivers who are engaged in caring for a disabled adult with communication and swallowing disorders. Most of these are conducted by other health professionals, but it will be helpful for speech-language pathologists and audiologists to gather preliminary information in order to develop a profile of any areas of concern. There are several categories of information that may be included in an initial intake:

- Background on the caregiver and the caregiving situation:
  - Relationship to patient
  - Where caregiving is conducted
  - Duration of caregiving
  - Other supportive persons in family network
  - Financial resources
  - Caregiver's employment status
- Caregiver's perception of health and status of patient:
  - Activities of daily living (ADLs) and instrumental activities of daily living (IADLs) performed without assistance
  - Medications administered
  - Language, speech, hearing, swallowing diagnosis
  - Memory loss or cognitive impairment
  - Motor or behavioral problems
- Caregiver values and preferences:
  - Willingness of caregiver to assume responsibilities of caregiving
  - Willingness of patient to accept care
  - Cultural issues that might impact care arrangements
- Well-being of the caregiver:
  - Health conditions or symptoms
  - Depression or other emotional factors (e.g. anxiety)
  - Perceived overall quality of life
  - Social outlets and other efforts to reduce stress
- Consequences of caregiving:
  - Financial strain
  - Family relationship strain
  - Problems with communicating with care recipient
- Use of outside resources to help with caregiving
- Caregiver skills/abilities/knowledge:
  - Caregiving confidence and competencies
  - Appropriate knowledge of communication or swallowing disorder
- Caregiver resources:
  - Caregiver network and perceived social support

- o Financial resources (health care and service benefits, entitlements such as Veterans Affairs, Medicare)
- o Community resources and services (caregiver support programs, religious organizations, volunteer agencies)

Assessments That Evaluate Impact on Caregivers

Once the case history is completed, the information can be shared with other professionals on the interdisciplinary team or in the referral network, for example, case managers, physicians, psychologists, social workers, and counselors. These professionals may then choose from a number of assessment instruments of caregiver strain, stress, coping, grief, and/or burden to complete their evaluations. Several can be accessed online. The formats vary from self-reporting assessments, interviews, or Internet interactive surveys. Most are paper and pencil assessments that capture the feelings of caregivers on dimensions of quality of life, life satisfaction, and feelings of control. Speech-language pathologists and audiologists should become familiar with these instruments, which include measurements of caregiver burden, coping, grief, strain, stress, and self-assessment and efficacy.

Measurements of Caregiver Burden

Caregiver Burden Inventory (Novak & Guest, 1989)

The Caregiver Burden Inventory measures caregiver burden as it relates to time, developmental comparison with peers, physical health, social relationships, and emotional health. This 19-item assessment uses a 5-point scale to measure four types of perceived burdens: time-dependence burden, developmental burden, physical burden, emotional burden, and social burden. The instrument is accessible at http://www.fullcirclecare.org/caregiver issues/health/burden.html

Caregiver Burden Scale
(Dumont, Fillion, Gagnon, & Bernier, 2008)

The Caregiver Burden Scale is an 18-item scale that measures stress perceived by the caregiver on a 4-point scale at the end of the care recipient's life.

Cost of Care Index (Kosberg & Cairl, 1986)

The Cost of Care Index measures different aspects of burden including personal and social restrictions, emotional health, worthiness of caregiving, relationship with care recipient, and economic costs. There are four items using 4-point scales for each: (a) personal and social restrictions, (b) physical and emotional health, (c) value investment in caregiving, and (d) perception of the care recipient as a provocateur.

Montgomery Burden Interview
(Montgomery, Gonyea, & Hooyman, 1985)

Two scales are used to assess both objective and subjective burden. The objective scale focuses on privacy, time, personal freedom, amount of money available, amount of energy, number of vacation and recreational activities, relationships with other family members, and health. The subjective scale focuses on attitudes and emotional reactions toward caregiving. There are nine items in the objective scale and 13 items in the subjective scale. Each scale uses a 5-point rating.

Novel Caregiver Burden
(Elmstahl, Malmberg, & Annerstedt, 1996)

This instrument measures strain, isolation, disappointment, and emotional involvement. There are 20 items and a 4-point scale.

Perceived Burden Scale (Poulshock & Deimling, 1984)

The Perceived Burden Scale measures the extent to which caregivers believe that changes have occurred because of problems or concerns encountered in caregiving. There are 22 items and a 5-point scale.

Perceived Caregiver Burden Scale
(Stommel, Given, & Given, 1990)

The Perceived Caregiver Burden Scale measures caregiver burden in terms of perceptions and feelings about caregivers' physical and emotional health, family relationships, social life, work, and finances. The instrument has 31 items and uses a 4-point scale.

Perceived Caregiver Burden Scale, Revised (Gupta, 1999)

Using 13 items and a 4-point scale, the Perceived Caregiver Burden Scale, Revised, is a shorter version of the Perceived Caregiver Burden Scale. This tool measures caregiver burden in terms of perceptions and feelings about caregivers' physical and emotional health, family relationships, social life, work, and finance.

Screen for Caregiver Burden (Vitaliano, Scanlan, Krenz, Schwartz, & Marcovina, 1996)

This instrument uses 25 items and a 5-point scale to measure objective and subjective burden relating to occurrence of care demands and distress associated with them.

Short Form Zarit Burden Interview (Bedard, Molloy, Squire, Duboid, Lever, & O'Donnell, 2001)

This is a shorter version of the Zarit Burden Interview designed to measure impact of caregiving. There are 12 items (5-point scale).

Zarit Burden Interview
(Zarit, Reever, & Bach-Peterson, 1980)

This widely used interview schedule measures caregiver appraisal of the impact of caregiving and burden related to health, psychological well-being, finances, social life, and relationship with the impaired person. There are 22 items and a 5-point scale. Items are summed to provide subscale scores. The assessment is readily available to the public and is translated in several languages, besides English: Hebrew, Spanish, Japanese, Turkish, French, Swedish, and Chinese. The instrument is readily available at http://rgps.on.ca/giic/GiiC/pdfs/Appendix%201%20-%20Zarit %20Burden%20Interview.pdf

Measure of Caregiver Coping

Brief COPE (Carver, 1997)

This assessment has 14 subscales and 28 items that assess specific coping responses to caregiving. The Brief COPE demonstrates high levels of reliability and validity and may be helpful to use when discussing the demands of caring for a disabled adult. The instrument is translated into Spanish, French, German, Greek, and Korean. All versions, including English, are accessible at http://www.psy.miami.edu/faculty/ccarver/CCscales.html

Measure of Caregiver Grief

Caregivers Grief Inventory-Short Form (Marwit & Meuser, 2005)

This is an 18-item inventory that measures caregiver grief during progressive disease. The instrument is also a reliable instrument for measuring grief that caregivers experience when a loved one has acquired a brain injury. The Caregivers Grief Inventory-Short Form is accessible at http://tadrc.wustl.edu/AboutUs/PDFs/ MM-CGI%20Short%20Form.pdf

Measures of Caregiving Strain

Caregiver Strain Index (CSI) (Robinson, 1983)

The CSI measures caregiver strain in 12 items using a 2-point scale. The purpose of the measurement is to probe for caregiver strain using yes/no response scales. The tool effectively identifies families who may benefit from more in-depth assessment and follow-up. A positive screen (seven or more items positive) on the CSI indicates a need for more in-depth assessment to facilitate appropriate intervention. The CSI may be accessed at http://consultgerirn.org/uploads/File/Caregiver%20Strain%20Index.pdf

Care-Related Strain (Whitlatch, Schur, Noelker, Ejaz, & Looman, 2001)

The Care-Related Strain measures the distress felt by a caregiver as a result of having a relative in a nursing home. There are seven items using a 4-point scale.

Family Strain Scale (Morycz, 1985)

The Family Strain Scale has five items that measure subjective burden related to emotional/psychological affect, changes in living in living patterns, and changes in relationships/health.

Measures of Strain (Bass & Bowman, 1990)

The Measures of Strain evaluates three domains: difficulty of caregiving (threat to family well-being), negative consequences of caregiving, and perceptions of negative consequences of caregiving on the family. There are eight items: three items for appraised difficulty of caregiving (4-point scale); three items for negative consequences of caregiving (2-point scale); and two items for perceptions of negative consequences of caregiving on the family (2-point scale).

Modified Caregiver Strain Index (MCSI)
(Thornton & Travis, 2003)

The MCSI is a tool that can be used to quickly screen for caregiver strain with long-term family caregivers. It has 13 questions that measure strain related to care provision. There is at least one item for each of the following major domains: financial, physical, psychological, social, and personal. This instrument can be used to assess individuals of any age who have assumed the caregiving role for an older adult. The MCSI is a more recent version of the Caregiver Strain Index (CSI) developed in 1983, and it was modified and developed in 2003 with a sample of 158 family caregivers providing assistance to older adults living in a community-based setting. Scoring is 2 points for each "yes" and 1 point for each "sometimes" response. The higher the score, the higher is the level of caregiver strain. The MCSI may be accessed online at http://consultgerirn.org/uploads/File/trythis/try_this_14.pdf

Measures of Caregiver Stress

Caregiver Distress Activities
(Pearlin, Mullan, Semple, & Skaff, 1990)

The Caregiver Distress Activities instrument measures the effort that the caregiver makes to minimize symptoms of stress brought on by caregiving. It has eight items and uses a 4-point scale.

Caregiver Stress Check (Alzheimer's Association, n.d.)

The Caregiver Stress Check is an 8-item self-reporting survey on areas of concern to caregivers. Provided is corresponding and interactive information on resources appropriate for caregivers of persons with dementia. This instrument can be accessed at http://www.alz.org/care/alzheimers-dementia-stress-check.asp

Caregiver Stress Effects (Deimling & Bass, 1986)

The Caregiver Stress Effects measures aspects of family life that are negatively affected by the caregiving role, as well as restrictions in caregiver activities as a result of the caregiving role. The instrument has eight items for negative changes in the care recipient (such as disruptive behavior), the caregiver, and family relationships. There are five items for restrictions in the caregivers' activities and independence.

Caregivers' Stress Scale (Pearlin et al., 1990)

The Caregivers' Stress Scale measures 15 domains: cognitive status, problematic behavior, overload, relational deprivation, family conflict, job-caregiving conflict, economic strains, role captivity, loss of self, caregiving competence, personal gain, management of situation, management of meaning, management of distress, and expressive support. This instrument contains a series of 15 scales and uses 3-, 4-, and 5-point rating scales.

Perceived Stress Scale
(Cohen, Kamarck, & Mermelstein, 1983)

This tool measures the degree to which situations are perceived as being stressful using 14 items and a 5-point scale. It is accessible at http://www.memic.unimaas.nl:8888/daisy/SMILE-CMS/300-SMILE/version/1/part/6/data/perceived_stress_scale.pdf?branch=main&language=default

Relatives' Stress Scale (Greene, Smith, Geardiner, & Timbury, 1982)

The Relatives' Stress Scale measures the reactions from caregivers by relatives of elderly patients living in the community. It uses a 5-point scale to focus on three domains: personal distress in relation to the care recipient, life upset as a result of caregiving, and negative feelings toward the care recipient.

Measures of Self-Assessment and Self-Efficacy

Caregiver Self-Assessment Questionnaire
(American Medical Association, 2012)

The Caregiver Self-Assessment Questionnaire is an 18-item, caregiver self-report measure, developed by the American Medical Association as a means of helping physicians (and other health professionals) to assess the stress levels of family caregivers accompanying chronically ill older adult patients to their medical visits. This self-assessment instrument has been found to be a valid and reliable instrument that allows caregiver respondents to rate themselves in the areas of emotional and physical health and conduct their own scoring (Epstein-Lubow, Gaudiano, Hinckley, Salloway, & Miller, 2010). Included with the assessment instrument are recommendations for self-referrals and a listing of resources with contact information. A simple scoring system allows family caregivers to score their own results and to determine whether or not they are highly stressed. The accompanying scoring sheet suggests that if they are highly stressed, they consider seeing a doctor for a check-up for themselves and reaching out for caregiver support services. The phone numbers and websites for several caregiver resources, including the Eldercare Locator, are listed. The questionnaire and scoring forms, available in English and Spanish versions, are downloadable for free at http://www.caregiverslibrary.org/Portals/0/Caringfor Yourself_CaregiverSelfAssessmentQuestionaire.pdf

Revised Scale for Caregiving Self-Efficacy (Steffen, McKibbin, Zeiss, Gallagher-Thompson, & Bandura, 2002)

The Revised Scale for Caregiving Self-Efficacy has 15 items within three subscales (self-efficacy for obtaining respite, responding to disruptive patient behaviors, and controlling upsetting thoughts about caregiving). Items are rated on a 0 to 100 scale for current beliefs, with the stem of "How confident are you that you . . . ," and with items such as "Can you ask a friend/family member to stay with _____ for a day when you need to see a doctor for yourself?" The three subscales show strong internal consistency and adequate test–retest reliability. Construct validity is supported by relationships between these three facets of perceived caregiving efficacy and depression, anxiety, anger, perceived social support, and criticism.

Commonly Used Assessments for Caregivers

Of the instruments described, eight assessments are most widely used by health professionals to assess caregiver perceptions of the effects of coping, burden, stress, and strain on their quality of life. As can be seen in Table 6–1, one instrument is interactive online and provides resource information depending on the responses (Caregiver Stress Check). One tool was developed by the American Medical Association to alert caregivers when they should seek medical attention for stress-related health disorders (Caregivers Self-Assessment Questionnaire). Three are available in several languages other than English (Brief Cope, Zarit Burden Scale, and the Caregivers Self-Assessment Questionnaire).

Table 6–1. Commonly Used Assessments for Family Caregivers

Assessment	Description	Availability
Brief COPE (Carver, 1997)	A 28-item scale that assesses specific coping responses and strategies	Available in six languages. http://www.psy.miami.edu/ faculty/ccarver/sclBrCOPE.html
Caregiver Burden Inventory (Novak & Guest, 1989)	A 19-item inventory to assess caregiver burden	http://www.fullcirclecare.org/ caregiverissues/health/burden .html
Caregiver Self-Assessment Questionnaire (American Medical Association, n.d.)	An 18-item self-report measurement of caregiver stress	Available in English and Spanish. http://www.caregiverslibrary. org/Portals/0/CaringforYour self_CaregiverSelfAssessment Questionaire.pdf
Caregiver Strain Index (CSI) (Robinson, 1983)	Measures caregiver strain using 12 items	http://consultgerirn.org/ uploads/File/Caregiver%20 Strain%20Index.pdf
Caregiver Stress Check (Alzheimer's Association, n.d.)	An eight-item inventory with interactive Web resources for caregiver stress	http://www.alz.org/care/ alzheimers-dementia-stress-check.asp
Modified Caregiver Strain Index (Onega, 2013)	13 questions screen for caregiver strain	http://consultgerirn.org/ uploads/File/trythis/try_ this_14.pdf
Perceived Stress Scale (Cohen, Kamarck, & Mermelstein, 1983)	Measures the degree to which situations are perceived as stressful using 14 items	http://www.mindgarden.com/ docs/PerceivedStressScale.pdf
Zarit Burden Interview (Zarit, Reever, & Peterson, 1980)	Uses 22 items to measure caregiver responses to caregiving impact	Available in eight languages. http://www.rgpc.ca/best/ GiiC%20Resources/GiiC/pdfs/ 3%20Caregiver%20Support%20-%20The%20Zarit%20Burden%20 Interview.pdf

Recommended Assessment for Use by Speech-Language Pathologists and Audiologists

The Brief COPE (Carver, 1997) was investigated by Hornaday, Shadden, DiBrezzo, and Power (2008). This is perhaps the only instrument that is documented as a recommended tool for speech-language pathologists and audiologists to measure caregiving impact. These researchers concluded that the Brief COPE was quick to administer, well researched, and should be an addition to professional toolkits. The Brief COPE is shown in Table 6–2.

Summary

Caregiving can have both positive and negative consequences for the physical and emotional health of caregivers. Caregivers may find that they are experiencing caregiver burden, difficulties with coping, grief, strain, or stress during the fulfillment of their responsibilities.

Speech-language pathologists and audiologists come in contact with family caregivers frequently while assessing and treating acutely or chronically ill adults with disorders of communication or swallowing. The focus has tended to be on the patient with communication disorders rather than on the caregivers, even in patient-centered therapy. Typically, family members and friends provide case history information about the patient and are included in intervention decisions in patient-centered treatment. However, family caregivers are themselves at risk for developing debilitating diseases, depression and other emotional problems, and caregiver burnout. It is appropriate for speech-language pathologists and audiologists to gather information about family caregivers as well as persons with disorders of communication, swallowing, and hearing as bases for further counseling and referral for other services. Caregivers who become overwhelmed by the demands of caring for others will be unable to help their loved ones physically or emotionally, keep appointments, manage carry-over of treatment goals, or encourage patients to participate in therapy and support groups.

Table 6–2. Brief COPE

Instructions	These items deal with ways you've been coping with the stress in your life since you found out you were going to have to have this operation. There are many ways to try to deal with problems. These items ask what you've been doing to cope with this one. Obviously, different people deal with things in different ways, but I'm interested in how you've tried to deal with it. Each item says something about a particular way of coping. I want to know to what extent you've been doing what the item says. How much or how frequently. Don't answer on the basis of whether it seems to be working or not—just whether or not you're doing it. Use these response choices. Try to rate each item separately in your mind from the others. Make your answers as true FOR YOU as you can.
Scoring	1 = I haven't been doing this at all.
	2 = I've been doing this a little bit.
	3 = I've been doing this a medium amount.
	4 = I've been doing this a lot.

1. I've been turning to work or other activities to take my mind off things. 1 2 3 4

2. I've been concentrating my efforts on doing something about the situation I'm in. 1 2 3 4

3. I've been saying to myself "this isn't real." 1 2 3 4

4. I've been using alcohol or other drugs to make myself feel better. 1 2 3 4

5. I've been getting emotional support from others. 1 2 3 4

6. I've been giving up trying to deal with it. 1 2 3 4

7. I've been taking action to try to make the situation better. 1 2 3 4

8. I've been refusing to believe that it has happened. 1 2 3 4

9. I've been saying things to let my unpleasant feelings escape. 1 2 3 4

10. I've been getting help and advice from other people. 1 2 3 4

continues

Table 6–2. *continued*

11. I've been using alcohol or other drugs to help me get through it.	1	2	3	4
12. I've been trying to see it in a different light, to make it seem more positive.	1	2	3	4
13. I've been criticizing myself.	1	2	3	4
14. I've been trying to come up with a strategy about what to do.	1	2	3	4
15. I've been getting comfort and understanding from someone.	1	2	3	4
16. I've been giving up the attempt to cope.	1	2	3	4
17. I've been looking for something good in what is happening.	1	2	3	4
18. I've been making jokes about it.	1	2	3	4
19. I've been doing something to think about it less, such as going to movies, watching TV, reading, daydreaming, sleeping, or shopping.	1	2	3	4
20. I've been accepting the reality of the fact that it has happened.	1	2	3	4
21. I've been expressing my negative feelings.	1	2	3	4
22. I've been trying to find comfort in my religion or spiritual beliefs.	1	2	3	4
23. I've been trying to get advice or help from other people about what to do.	1	2	3	4
24. I've been learning to live with it.	1	2	3	4
25. I've been thinking hard about what steps to take.	1	2	3	4
26. I've been blaming myself for things that happened.	1	2	3	4
27. I've been praying or meditating.	1	2	3	4
28. I've been making fun of the situation.	1	2	3	4

Source: Carver, C. S. (1997). You want to measure coping but your protocol's too long: Consider the Brief COPE. *International Journal of Behavioral Medicine, 4,* 92–100. Retrieved from http://www.psy.miami.edu/faculty/ccarver/sclBrCOPE.html

There are a number of caregiver assessment instruments that are available and accessible. Eight are widely used by other health professionals to measure caregiver status. One tool, the Brief COPE (Carver, 1997) is translated into several languages and is recommended for use by speech-language pathologists and audiologists. The results of this assessment may be used to begin the conversations with caregivers about their needs and to refer them to other professionals when the intense responsibilities of caregiving are having negative effects on their health.

The Brief COPE is recommended to become part of the professional toolkit for speech-language pathologists and audiologists. Counseling within the scope of practice and referrals to appropriate professionals are the next steps.

References

Alzheimer's Association. (n.d.). *Alzheimer's stress check.* Retrieved from http://www.alz.org/care/alzheimers-dementia-stress-check.asp

American Medical Association. (2012). *Caregivers self-assessment questionnaire.* Retrieved from http://www.caregiverslibrary.org/Portals/0/CaringforYourself_CaregiverSeAssessmentQuestionaire.pdf

Bass, D. M., & Bowman, K. (1990). The transition from caregiving to bereavement: The relationship of care-related strain and adjustment to death. *Gerontologist, 31,* 32–42.

Bedard, M., Molloy, D. W., Squire, L., Dubois, S., Lever, J. A., & O'Donnell, M. (2001). The Zarit Burden Interview: A new short version and screening version. *Gerontologist, 41,* 652–657.

Carver, C. S. (1997). You want to measure coping but your protocol's too long: Consider the Brief COPE. *International Journal of Behavioral Medicine, 4,* 92–100.Census 2000 Special Report. (2005). *Disability and American families.* Retrieved from http://www.census.gov/prod/2005pubs/censr-23.pdf

Center on Aging Society. (2005). *How do family caregivers fare? A closer look at their experiences.* Data Profile, Number 3. Washington, DC: Georgetown University.

Cohen, S., Kamarck, T., & Mermelstein, R. (1983). A global measure of perceived stress. *Journal of Health and Social Behavior, 24,* 385–396.

Deimling, G. T., & Bass, D. M. (1986). Symptoms of mental impairment among elderly adults and their effects on family caregivers. *Journal of Gerontology, 41,* 778–784.

Dumont, S., Fillion, L., Gagnon, P., & Bernier, N. (2008). A new tool to assess family caregiver burden during end-of-life care. *Journal of Palliative Care, 24*(3), 151–161.

Elmstahl, S., Malmberg, B., & Annerstedt, L. (1996). Caregiver's burden of patients 3 years after stroke assessed by a Novel Caregiver Burden Scale. *Archives of Physical Medicine and Rehabilitation, 77,* 177–182.

Epstein-Lubow, G., Gaudiano, B. A., Hinckley, M., Salloway, S., & Miller, I. W. (2010). Evidence for the validity of the American Medical Association's Caregiver Self-Assessment Questionnaire as a screening measure for depression. *Journal of the American Geriatrics Society, 58*(2), 387–388.

Family Caregiver Alliance. (2012). *Grief.* Retrieved from http://www. caregiver.org/caregiver/jsp/content_node.jsp?nodeid=404

Feinberg, L., & Houser, A. (2012). *Assessing family caregiver needs: Policy and practice considerations.* Washington, DC: AARP Public Policy Institute.

Feinberg, L., Reinhard, S. C., Houser, A., & Choula, R. (2012). *Valuing Invaluable: 2011 update. The growing contributions and costs of family caregiving.* Retrieved from http://assets.aarp.org/rgcenter/ ppi/ltc/i51-caregiving.pdf

Greene, J. G., Smith, R., Geardiner, M., & Timbury, C. C. (1982). Measuring behavioral disturbance of elderly demented patients and its effects on relatives: A factor analytic study. *Age and Ageing, 11,* 121–126.

Gupta, R. (1999). The Revised Caregiver Burden Scale: A preliminary evaluation. *Research on Social Work Practice, 4,* 508–520.

Hornaday, K., Shadden, B., DiBrezzo, R., & Powers, M. (2008). *Measuring coping in caregivers: Methodological challenges.* Research poster session presented at the Annual Convention of the American Speech-Language-Hearing Association, Chicago, IL.

Kosberg, J. I., & Cairl, R. E. (1986). The Cost of Care Index: A case management tool for screening informal care providers. *Gerontologist, 26,* 273–278.

Marwit, S. J., & Meuser, T. M. (2005). Development of a short form inventory to assess grief in caregivers of dementia patients. *Death Studies, 3,* 191–205.

Montgomery, R., Gonyea, J. G., & Hooyman, N. R. (1985). Caregiving and the experience of subjective and objective burden. *Family Relations, 34,* 19–26.

Morycz, R. K. (1985). Caregiving strain and the desire to institutionalize family members with Alzheimer's disease: Possible predictors and model development. *Research on Aging, 7,* 329–361.

Novak, M., & Guest, C. (1989). Application of a multidimensional Caregiver Burden Inventory. *Gerontologist, 29*, 798–803.

Onega, L. L. (2013). *The Modified Caregiver Strain Index (MCSI)*. Retrieved from http://consultgerirn.org/uploads/File/trythis/try_this_14.pdf

Pearlin, L. I., Mullan, J. T., Semple, S. J., & Skaff, M. M. (1990). Caregiving and the stress process: An overview of concepts and their measures. *Gerontologist, 30*, 583–594.

Poulshock, S. W., & Deimling, G. T. (1984). Families caring for elders in residence: Issues in the measurement of burden. *Journal of Gerontology, 39*, 230–239.

Robinson, B. C. (1983). Validation of a caregiver strain index. *Journal of Gerontology, 38*, 344–348.

Spillers, R. L., Wellisch, D. K., Kim, Y., Matthews, B. A., & Baker, F. (2008). Family caregivers and guilt in the context of cancer care. *Psychosomatics, 49*, 511–519. Retrieved from http://www.ncbi.nlm.nih.gov/pubmed/19122128

Steffen, A. M., McKibbin, C., Zeiss, A. M., Gallagher-Thompson, D. & Bandura, A. (2002). The revised scale for caregiving self-efficacy: Reliability and validity studies. *Journals of Gerontology: Psychological Sciences, 57*, 74–86.

Stommel, M., Given, C. W., & Given, B. (1990). Depression as an overriding variable explaining caregiver burdens. *Journal of Aging and Health, 2*, 81–102.

Thornton, M., & Travis, S. S. (2003). Analysis of the reliability of the Modified Caregiver Strain Index. *Journal of Gerontology, Series B, Psychological Sciences and Social Sciences, 58*, S127–S132.

Vitaliano, P. P., Scanlan, J. M., Krenz, C., Schwartz, R. S., & Marcovina, S. M. (1996). Psychological distress, caregiving, and metabolic variables. *Journals of Gerontology, 51B*(5), P290–P297.

Whitlatch, C. J., Schur, D., Noelker, L. S., Ejaz, F. K., & Looman, W. J. (2001). The stress process of family caregiving in institutional settings. *Gerontologist, 41*, 462–473.

Zarit, S. H., Reever, K. E., & Bach-Peterson, J. (1980). Relatives of the impaired elderly: Correlates of feelings of burden. *Gerontologist, 20*, 649–655.

7

Educating and Counseling Caregivers Within the Clinical Setting

Joan C. Payne

Jungbauer, Döll, and Wilz (2008) found that caregivers have differing needs at different points of caregiving. During the initial, acute hospitalization period, caregivers may desire more detailed information about the nature of the disease or illness. During the outpatient rehabilitation period, caregivers may need more emotional assistance.

It is clear that speech-language pathologists and audiologists have critical roles in providing information and emotional assistance to persons with communication disorders and their families. Several important texts speak to providing preferred methods for education and counseling within the scopes of practice (Flasher & Fogle, 2012; DiLollo & Neimeyer, 2014;

Holland, 2007; Holland & Nelson, 2014; Tanner, 2003, 2008). The emphasis of these writings is on the patient with the communication disorder. A common theme is how to best provide education and support to patients and their families who are struggling to understand communication disorders and the behavioral, psychological, and motor changes in the patient because of disabling conditions.

This chapter differs from that of others in that the focus is on the family caregiver who provides for the person with the communication disorder. It is argued that caregivers, as much as persons with disorders of communication and swallowing, are in need of sustained intervention to help them adjust and thrive within the context of caregiving. It is argued, also, that speech-language pathologists and audiologists can support family caregivers within the scope of practice through education/training, emotional assistance, and referrals to other professionals.

Two important constructs should guide clinicians to educate and counsel caregivers from the American Speech-Language-Hearing Association (ASHA) and the American Academy of Audiology (AAA). One is the *Code of Ethics* (ASHA, 2010r), which asserts that "Individuals shall use every resource, including referral when appropriate, to ensure that high-quality service is provided." Another is the corpus of policy statements on practice guidelines for speech-language pathologists and audiologists such as *Preferred Practice Patterns for the Profession of Speech-Language Pathology* (ASHA, 2004b), *Preferred Practice Patterns for the Profession of Audiology* (ASHA, 2006), *Scope of Practice in Speech-Language Pathology* (ASHA, 2007), *Scope of Practice in Audiology* (ASHA, 2004a), *Guidelines for Audiologists Providing Informational and Adjustment Counseling to Families of Infants and Young Children with Hearing Loss Birth to 5 Years of Age* (ASHA, 2008), and *Standards of Practice for Audiologists* (AAA, 2012).

For speech-language pathologists, it is affirmed that "educating and providing in-service training to families, caregivers, and other professionals" are within the acceptable scope of practice (ASHA, 2007). Specifically, educating caregivers to work with persons with disabling and chronic conditions that disrupt communication and swallowing should become a major focus of the educational and training process. While family caregivers are not specifically named as candidates for counseling, practitioners are enjoined within scope of practice policy statements to consider the personal and social contexts of their patients. These contexts can and should include the functioning and well-being of caregivers upon whom the patient is dependent for around-the-clock care and, indeed, survival.

In addition, ASHA (2004a) mandates that audiologists should, "provide comprehensive services to individuals with normal hearing who interact with persons with a hearing impairment." AAA (2012) goes further to say that audiologists should, where appropriate, develop a plan that enables family members to care for the hearing impaired individual. Perhaps *Guidelines for Audiologists Providing Informational and Adjustment Counseling to Families of Infants and Young Children with Hearing Loss Birth to 5 Years of Age* (ASHA, 2008) is the most comprehensive and definitive policy statement regarding family caregivers of persons with communication disorders. See Appendix A for these guidelines. In this statement, the family is recognized as a critical source of support, information, and advocacy. There is the compassionate recognition that clinicians should provide both informational and adjustment counseling to family caregivers because of the importance of their roles in assisting their loved ones. The rationale is that individuals with a communication disorder, and in this case, a hearing disorder, are reliant on the physical, mental, and emotional health of those providing care for their acceptance of and adjustment to the communication disorder. There is also the recognition that family caregivers are themselves in need of emotional and other forms of support as they struggle to cope with often difficult diagnoses. Although not intended for caregivers of mature adults, the philosophy undergirding this policy statement has relevance for family caregivers of disabled persons across the life span. Both education and counseling are deemed as equally important strategies for family caregivers. That is, "For counseling to be most effective, information counseling and adjustment counseling/emotional support must be balanced. The goal is to facilitate the development of informed, independent, and empowered families who will make good decisions."

Fundamentals of Family Caregiver Education

Developing a Plan of Education and Training

Caregivers frequently complain that they really do not understand what has happened to their family member or friend, or how they can improve their communication interactions. Clinicians may prioritize the patient's disorder over the caregiver's concerns because of time restrictions. Hence, a caregiver's need to understand a communication disorder or how to communicate with an impaired adult may not be fully addressed because of the nature or severity of the patient's disorder. As a result, professionals may be less available to assist a caregiver with how to manage breakdowns in communication outside of the clinical setting.

However, assisting a caregiver to increase ability and knowledge has been shown to produce positive short-term results in interactions between the caregiver and care recipient (Holland & Nelson, 2014; Sörenson, Pinquart, & Duberstein, 2002). There are many opportunities to educate caregivers when a person is referred for speech-language pathology or audiology services. As a major part of their education, caregivers can be trained on how to communicate more effectively with their loved ones.

Before starting a program of education, clinicians should determine what each caregiver already knows and then supply whatever information is missing, avoiding medical terms and jargon as much as possible (Payne, 2014). Answers to questions about what a caregiver understands about communication and swallowing, the type of disorder the patient has, and the role of the speech-language pathologist or audiologist in treating the communication or swallowing disorder can be used to guide an education/training program.

Both verbal and written information should be shared with caregivers. Clinicians should develop an easily understood oral and written description that gives information about health disorder(s) and the effects on communication and swallowing. Clinicians can also use free or low-cost educational materials to explain chronic and disabling conditions and how these compromise all areas of communication and swallowing. Many of these materials are appropriate for a multicultural, multilingual audience and are available from advocacy organizations, such as ASHA, AARP, the Alzheimer's Association, the American Heart Association, and the American Cancer Association, among others.

Training/Educating in Speech-Language Pathology

Breakdowns in interpersonal communication between a caregiver and a care recipient can make their daily interactions extremely frustrating. This frustration increases stress and burden and significantly alters family relations. With the help of the speech-language pathologist, caregivers can be trained to use strategies to avoid misunderstandings. Mason-Baughman and Lander (2012), for example, found that training caregivers of persons with dementia to use communication strategies and aids lessened their feelings of frustration and isolation. According to these researchers, the speech-language pathologist can serve as an educator for family members and caregivers, as well as provide direct intervention and support for individuals with dementia. They report that the speech-language pathologist-led training was more effective than even caregiver-friendly literature. Training sessions led by the speech-language pathologist which featured simple language, functional explanations, visual materials and games, and information on the potential benefits of the strategies, encouraged caregivers to use some of the strategies.

Education/Training in Audiology

Educating caregivers to identify solutions to behavioral disorders and hearing loss associated with some chronic diseases can also prove to be helpful in reducing caregiver stress. In an article by Palmer, Adams, Bourgeois, Durrant, and Rossi (1999), eight persons with Alzheimer's disease and behavioral problems were fitted with hearing aids. These researchers reported significant reductions in negative behaviors after the fittings and appropriate aural rehabilitation.

Another exemplar of training comes from research on fear of falling (FoF) which can be devastating for older persons and their caregivers. Educating caregivers on the factors in hearing and balance that cause FoF can make a positive difference in the quality of life for both the caregiver and the care recipient. Vestibular rehabilitation involving caregivers and patients can result in lifestyle changes that reduce FoF and improve patients' balance confidence (Honaker & Kretschmer, 2014).

Fundamentals of Counseling for Family Caregivers

According to Flasher and Fogle (2012), counseling within the professionals of speech-language pathology and audiology is an applied social science and a "helping, interpersonal relationship in which the clinician's intentions are to assist a person or family member to understand a communication or swallowing disorder . . . as well as ways to cope with these disorders" (p. 4). It should be emphasized that the focus of family caregiver counseling should be to address the caregiver's needs by creating a "safe harbor" in which there can be a sharing of personal concerns freely and confidentially. This can only occur if trust has been established (Holland & Nelson, 2014).

Once education and caregiver training are completed, it will be important to assist caregivers with the means to identify the kind of emotional support they need at various stages of their caregiving (Holland, 2007; Raina et al., 2004). As a starting point, the results of a caregiver interview such as the *Brief COPE* (Carver, 2007) described in Chapter 6 can be used to begin a conversation about emotional needs.

Importantly, the clinician as a compassionate listener must not interject personal biases into the listening process. Other guidelines suggested by DiLollo and Neimeyer (2014) and Holland and Nelson (2014) are as follows:

- Counseling can be brief and as simple as a conversation.
- Counseling should be directed to the level of meaning rather than only behavior or rational thought.
- Counseling should include strategies for meaningful action in order for change to occur.

- Within counseling, effective solutions are needed that facilitate optimal functioning and engagement.
- Attention to details are required even if they appear to be outside of the current situation.
- Counseling should incorporate perceptiveness and an attitude of respect of sensitivity and respect in every aspect of the clinical encounter.

A caregiver may be at one of three stages of emotional need or a combination of stages. McIntyre (2012) provides insight into three stages of emotional need that caregivers may experience while caring for a person during the course of a chronic or acute illness:

1. Early Stage: What is happening or what has happened to my loved one? (Caregiver reactions: surprise, fear, denial, confusion, sadness)
2. Middle Stage: How long does this last? (Caregiver reactions: frustration, guilt, resentment, conflicting demands)
3. Late Stage: How do I respect the needs of my loved one? (Caregiver reactions: sadness, guilt, surrender, regret, relief, solace, closure)

Clinicians should pay close attention to where a caregiver is in these stages. The question of professional boundaries in counseling lies between the caregiver's needs, the clinician's scope of practice, and the professional Code of Ethics. How these factors intersect is in the clinician's ability to adhere to professional boundaries while still affirming the emotional reactions to caregiving experienced by the caregiver (Harvard Medical College, 2012). Another approach is to direct caregivers to appropriate sources of information. For many, having one's own emotions validated as well as having appropriate and needed caregiver resources may significantly decrease anxiety and strain.

There may be other areas of emotional need that require counseling outside of the sphere of speech-language pathology and audiology. Flasher and Fogle (2012) suggest that a challenge to professional boundaries is when we must make decisions about whether we are equipped to provide service to a particular client. They go further to give examples of issues beyond the scope of practice in speech-language pathology and audiology, including such topics as chronic depression, legal conflicts, marital problems, elder abuse, and chemical dependence.

Developing a Program of Counseling

Emotional needs may be supported, in part, by the clinician's acknowledgment that the caregiver's questions and emotions are legitimate reactions to difficult and intense situations. Clinicians can suggest alternative ways to cope with stress. Thompson and his colleagues (1993), for example, noted that caregivers report that they find pleasurable activities with family and friends to be the most productive in lightening caregiver burden. Other forms of emotional assistance for caregivers within the speech-language pathology and audiology clinical setting can include the following:

- Compassionate listening
- Suggestions for de-stressing (massages, aromatics, music, herbal teas, time with family and friends, exercise, yoga)
- Relaxation techniques
- Photonovelas (fotonovelas)

The photonovela (fotonovela) uses photographs and script to make complicated health information simpler and more user-friendly for caregivers (Martinez, 2008). It is particularly helpful for those whose primary language is not English or who have limited reading literacy. The advantage of the photonovela is that the pictures and script can be customized in different languages and in the ethnic representation of persons. The effectiveness of this tool was demonstrated by Gallagher-Thompson and her associates (2015) who found that Hispanic American caregivers of persons with dementia reported less depressive symptoms when using a photonovela to help them cope with their care recipients' condition. Moreover, the researchers found that Hispanic American caregivers relied more on the information from the photonovela than from information given in the usual format. This pictorial tool can be adapted for any linguistic or ethnic group or disorder and can be used to explain how the caregiver can engage in self-care or how to manage caregiving responsibilities more effectively.

Within the clinician's scope of practice, also, is sharing resource information about communication disorders (Chapters 4 and 5) and resource websites designed specifically for caregivers that encourages them to examine options for addressing their concerns. This information can lead to a discussion about referrals to professionals in other areas of expertise.

Many caregivers are ill-prepared for caregiving and have numerous issues to resolve in order to provide optimal care. Some issues are directly related to help with the communication disorder of the care recipient and can be addressed by the speech-language pathologist or audiologist. However, other issues relate to the caregivers' own health and well-being, and still others are related to the caregiver's need for resources that can provide relief, closure, or assistance, such as

- health insurance;
- caregiver resources;
- income;
- housing options;
- support groups;
- transportation;
- meals;
- respite care;
- financial literacy;
- adult day care;
- health care practitioners;
- legal services (wills, power of attorney, advanced directives);
- veterans benefits;
- hospice care;
- home health care providers;
- estate planning;
- grief/bereavement counseling; and
- home safety.

Table 7–1 provides information on websites that can be readily accessed to provide answers to some of the concerns that caregivers may have. The information on these sites can be shared and discussed with caregivers during counseling.

Table 7–1. Caregiver Concerns and Informational Websites

Caregiver Concern	Possible Solution(s)
Insurance	Medicare: http://www.medicare.gov
	Centers for Medicaid and Medicare: http://www.cms.gov/Medicare-Medicaid-Coordination/Medicare-and-Medicaid-Coordination/Medicare-Medicaid-Coordination-Office
	Sites provide information on Medicaid and Medicare benefits and private insurance.
Caregiver resources	Administration on Community Living (U.S. Department of Health and Human Services, DHHS). Includes:
	Alzheimers.gov—This site is the government's resource for Alzheimer's and related dementias.
	Eldercare Locator—The ACL Eldercare Locator is a website and call center that links to state and local agencies on aging and community-based organizations that serve older adults and their caregivers.
	The Benefits Check Up website helps consumers find benefits programs that help them pay for prescription drugs, health care, rent, utilities, and other needs. The website includes information from more than 1,650 public and private benefits programs from all 50 states and Washington DC.
	Helpful Publications and Website Resources—A part of the Eldercare Locator website, there are useful topic-specific resources for older adults, caregivers, and aging professionals.
	Long-Term Care Planning—Long-term care includes a variety of services and supports to meet health or personal care needs over an extended period of time. The National Clearinghouse for Long-Term Care Information website provides information and resources to help individuals plan for future long-term care. http://www.acl.gov/Get_Help/Help_Older_Adults/Index.aspx

Table 7–1. *continued*

Caregiver Concern	Possible Solution(s)
Income	U.S. Office of Social Security Administration—Explains benefits related to retirement, disability, Medicare, and Supplemental Security Income (SSI) and provides online applications for benefits. Free interpreter services are available. Other languages available for online reading are American Sign Language, Arabic, Armenian, Chinese, Farsi, Italian, Korean, French, Greek, Haitian Creole, Hmong, Tagalog, Somali, Polish, Spanish, Portugese, Russian, and Vietnamese. http://www.ssa.gov
Housing	HELPGUIDE.org—Explains options for senior house: (a) aging in place; (b) village concept; (c) National Occurring Retirement Communities (NORC); (d) independent living; (e) assisted living; and (f) nursing homes. http://www.helpguide.org/elder/senior_housing_residential_care_types.htm
Support Groups	Alzheimer's—http://www.alz.org
	American Heart—http://www.aha.org
	American Cancer—http://www.cancer.org
	ALS—http://www.alsa.org
	MS—http://www.nationalmssociety.org
	Lewy Body Dementia—http://www.lbda.org
	Parkinson's disease—http://www.pdf.org
Transportation	Local churches
	Local mass transit
	State offices on aging
Meals	Meals on Wheels Association of America http://www.mowaa.org
Respite care	Alzheimer's and Dementia Caregiver Center—Defines respite care and describes types of respite care. Provides links to home care, adult day care centers, and residential care facilities. http://www.alz.org

continues

Table 7–1. *continued*

Caregiver Concern	Possible Solution(s)
Financial literacy	AARP—Provides information on managing finances and avoiding scams. http://www.aarp.org
	National Council on Aging—Provides information to professionals for workshops on financial management and avoiding scams, including PowerPoint presentations. http://www.ncoa.org/enhance-economic-security/economic-security-Initiative/savvy-saving-seniors/
Adult day care	Local Alzheimer's Association office
	Local AARP office
Health care	Healthgrades provides names, specialties, contact information, and patient ratings for physicians, dentists, and hospitals by state. Includes geriatricians. http://www.healthgrades.com
Legal services	National Legal Resource Center (Administration on Aging) has valuable information and links to legal help for older adults and for advocates as well. http://www.nlrc.aoa.gov
	National Academy of Elder Law Attorneys has members who help seniors with legal issues; there is a list of attorneys on their website. http://www.naela.org
	Legal Services Corporation Directory contains a nationwide directory of attorneys and judges who help low-income older adults in civil (not criminal) matters. http://www.lsc.gov
	National Disability Rights Network has a directory of disability rights agencies nationwide. http://www.ndrn.org
	American Bar Association provides useful links to lawyer referral services and pro bono legal help for those with limited incomes. http://www.americanbar.org

Table 7–1. *continued*

Caregiver Concern	Possible Solution(s)
Legal services *continued*	National Bar Association—The nation's oldest and largest national association of predominantly African American lawyers and judges, with affiliate chapters throughout the United States. http://www.nationalbar.org
	Hispanic National Bar Association—Largest national association of predominantly Hispanic lawyers. http://www.hnba.com
Veteran's benefits	Veterans Administration—Provides information on disability compensation, pensions, and health benefits. http://benefits.va.gov/benefits
Hospice care	Hospice Care of America site has important information on organizations that provide hospice care and reading materials on hospice care and bereavement. http://hospicecareofamerica.com/resources.html
Home health care	Medicare.gov—Explains home health services, how to arrange for home health services, and what Medicare Parts A and B will cover, including speech-language pathology services. http://www.medicare.gov/what-medicare-covers/home-health-care/home-health-care-what-is-it-what-to-expect.html
Estate planning	ElderLawAnswers has been the Web's leading online destination for reader-friendly news and explanations of Medicaid coverage of long-term care, Medicare benefits, estate planning, guardianship, and other legal issues affecting seniors. Access to a nationwide network of prescreened attorneys who focus their practices on helping the elderly. http://www.elderlawanswers.com/about-us

continues

Table 7–1. *continued*

Caregiver Concern	Possible Solution(s)
Grief/ bereavement	Family Caregiver Alliance (National Center on Caregiving)—Site provides information about causes and symptoms of grief and bereavement and provides other websites where caregivers can find grief counselors in their communities. Site also recommends readings on grief and bereavement.
	https://www.caregiver.org/grief-and-loss
Safety	National Safety Council—Site gives information on preventing falls and fall-proofing the home. http://www.nsc.org/safety_home/ HomeandRecreationalSafety/Falls/Pages/ OlderAdultFalls.aspx
	U.S. Food and Drug Administration—Medication interactions are discussed as well as medication safety tips for older adults.
	http://www.fda.gov/ForConsumers/ ConsumerUpdates/ucm399834.htm
	National Fire Protection Association—Tips on protecting the safety of older adults in a home fire.
	http://www.nfpa.org/safety-information/ for-consumers/populations/older-adults
	Medical Alert Systems—Lifefone and Life Alert are two well-recognized systems for ensuring that older adults can call for assistance (Emergency, fire, police) if alone at home. Others, like ADT, also have medical alert systems for seniors.
	LifeFone: http://www.lifefone.com/?mm_campaign= 3648d65c0712f5bcad17506602a41fb3&keyword=el derly%20home%20safety&utm_source=Google&utm_ medium=CPC&utm_campaign=Alert-Safety&gclid= Cj0KEQjw3cKeBRDG-KKqqIj4qJgBEiQAOamX_ WnKlt2InHSzfkyO-BMfmIrwQMca6rRm-ImnfBsc 6MMaAvmW8P8HAQ
	LifeAlert: http://www.lifealerthelp.com/?gclid= Cj0KEQjw3cKeBRDG-KKqqIj4qJgBEiQAOamX_Ukupgo bgdiLSnDrFiCctzUQDYTr39IVhDUWvNZ20pQaAolh8 P8HAQ
	ADT: http://www.adt.com/media/health/

Making Referrals

Some caregivers may need more intensive and hands-on support for emotional, mental, and physical concerns. It is appropriate to refer to other professionals when a caregiver's needs are greater than the experience, training, and certification of the speech-language pathologist or audiologist. Under the Rules of Ethics (ASHA, 2010r), "Individuals shall use every resource, including referral when appropriate, to ensure that high-quality service is provided." because, "Individuals shall engage in only those aspects of the professions that are within the scope of their professional practice and competence, considering their level of education, training, and experience" (ASHA, 2010r).

Another perspective is that clinicians are working within the scope of practice by "providing referrals and information to other professionals, agencies, and/or consumer organizations" (ASHA, 2007). Similarly, audiologists are reminded that rehabilitation should also include, "Availability of counseling relating to psycho social aspects of hearing loss, and other auditory dysfunction, and processes to enhance communication competence" as well as, "Skills training and consultation concerning environmental modifications to facilitate development of receptive and expressive communication" (ASHA, 2004a).

Supporting Multicultural Caregivers

As discussed in Chapter 3, caregivers have differing views on caregiving because of cultural norms and expectations. In addition, diverse caregivers have differences in worldviews which have to be considered and respected in order to establish trust and engage in effective counseling. Some general guidelines may be helpful for assisting caregivers in a culturally sensitive and competent manner. The guidelines suggested by Payne and Wright-Harp (2014) are adapted for caregivers:

- Provide health communication that is clear, easy to understand, in the patient's language, and reflective of the communication context of the patient.

- o Use written materials that reflect ethnic diversity.
- o Use text material that is easy to read and in the patient's language.
- o Provide verbal information through an interpreter.
- o Tailor messages to the context of the caregiver, whether high context (nonverbal communication and silence are valued) or low context (spoken and written communication are valued).
- o Avoid cultural faux-pas—using the caregiver's first name, telling jokes, or asking for personal information before trust has been established.
- Respect divergent views on health and wellness.
  - o Ask the caregiver to describe his or her views on how caregiving is affecting his or her life and health.
  - o Become informed about how health care decisions, including physical and mental health, are made in the caregiver's community.
  - o Be aware of how differences in coping styles vary within cultures and are often tied to religion among some cultures.
- Respect differences in family structures.
  - o Be mindful that there is no model of the perfect family caregiver.
  - o Understand that, in some cultures, families are largely patriarchal; in others, the eldest member speaks for the family; in still others, families are matriarchal or multigenerational; these arrangements work for the families involved.
  - o Accept that cultural norms for filial piety and caregiver obligation govern who has the major responsibility for caregiving.
- Respect divergent views on time and personal space.
  - o Consider that time is relative and meaningful in different ways in different cultures.
  - o Respect that use of personal space is culture driven and that there are cultural variations in how personal and social space are defined.
  - o Understand that in some religions, personal space is delineated according to gender and/or marital status.

- Respect divergent views of health care.
  - Know that cultures differ in the ways that illness is explained and in what is acceptable to hear about illness.
  - Know, also, that some caregivers accept caregiving responsibilities more cheerfully than others.
- Respect language differences.
  - Provide a translator for caregivers whose primary language is not English.
  - Appreciate that one's language is a deeply personal aspect of culture.
- Respect other views of the responsibilities of caregiving.
  - Be knowledgeable that in some cultures, the work necessary to provide care is viewed differently.
  - Understand that caregiving in some communities may be defined by parameters other than blood relations.
- Respect the family caregivers' autonomy in decision making.
  - With the permission of the caregiver, include all members of the extended family in counseling.
  - Validate the opinions of the family caregiver.
  - Do not presume that the family caregiver has no knowledge of communication disorders; interview the family on this issue and build from there.
- Respect differences in emotional expression.
  - Be aware that a smile does not necessarily mean agreement; it sometimes means confusion or respect.
  - Do not be offended by differences in how a caregiver can look the clinician in the eyes.
- One size does not fit all.
  - Tailor counseling to the caregiver's needs.
  - Provide support and information on resources in the family's preferred community.

Additional guidelines for counseling diverse cultural and ethnic caregivers are given in Table 7–2. As can be seen, there may be different expectations for working with diverse caregivers. The expectations are given by ethnic group.

Table 7–2. Expectations for Culturally Diverse Caregivers

Ethnic Group	Expectations
Non-Hispanic Whites	Expect that caregivers will be assertive about counseling needs and will communicate verbally well. Expect, also, that caregivers will confront the clinician if their views are not in agreement. Expect limited physical contact but direct eye contact.
African Americans	Expect that it will take time to establish a bond of trust necessary for the caregiver to reveal personal information. Respect is important. Address caregivers by titles: Mr., Mrs., or Ms., and last name until given permission to use first name. Expect that caregivers use an emotive approach to handling caregiver stress rather than an analytic approach. Expect that religion occupies an important role in handling caregiver responsibilities.
Hispanic Americans	Expect that Hispanic women, in particular, are likely to view caregiver burdens as "God's will." Counseling may be viewed as an option solely for the lazy or inept. Expect that short-term, time-limited counseling that focuses on current problems and solutions is preferable than long-term counseling.
Native Americans/ Alaska Natives	Expect caregivers to react in a passive manner until trust is established. Passivity may be used to avoid revealing personal information and silence may mean that the caregiver disagrees with the clinician.
Asian American/ Pacific Islanders	Expect to build an interpersonal relationship and establish trust. Caregivers may be extremely reluctant to share personal information. Expect to take on an authoritative manner to build confidence and trust. Expect to give directives in counseling rather than "talk therapy."
Middle Eastern Americans (Muslims)	Expect to assign same-sex counselors whenever possible. Expect that women may defer to husbands and that the husband may answer questions addressed to his wife. Avoid direct eye contact with members of the opposite sex, particularly from female to male. Personal problems are usually taken care of within the family; caregivers may be reluctant to engage in counseling. Negative information should be presented with great care and in stages.

Sources: Carteret (2011); Payne (2014); Payne and Wright-Harp (2014); and Salas-Provance (2012).

When to Refer

When a caregiver's concerns are outside of the scope of practice for speech-language pathologists and audiologists, it is important to know when to refer and which professional or community service is appropriate. The best time to refer is as soon as there is an indication that caregivers are having difficulties in coping with their responsibilities or when there are major changes in the care environment across a continuum of acute care, rehabilitation or outpatient care, institutional care, or community re-entry (Cameron & Cignac, 2008).

Considerations for Referrals

Making appropriate referrals includes being aware of the cultural sensitivities of persons needing specialized counseling. For example, although a heterogeneous group, African American caregivers are more likely to accept referrals if they feel that the counselors are culturally aware and respectful. These caregivers are also more inclined to look favorably upon community or church-based resources for counseling rather than professionals outside of their communities. Asian American and non-Hispanic white caregivers may feel equally comfortable with professionals who provide counseling both within and outside of the community, whereas Hispanic and Middle Eastern caregivers may prefer that the entire family be involved in counseling that is conducted in their preferred languages. For Muslims, counselors who are cognizant of their religious traditions will be preferable to counselors who are not. American Indian/Alaska Native caregivers may be more comfortable with counseling professionals who respect and appreciate their tribal traditions.

Ideally, clinicians should assess, educate, and recommend resources as part of the initial and subsequent discussions with family caregivers. However some caregivers may show early or consistent signs of being overwhelmed with caregiving responsibilities and may need expedited referrals. Some signs that a caregiver may need immediate referral assistance are as follows:

- Chronic lateness or consistently missing appointments
- Somatic complaints: not sleeping well or at all, not eating, experiencing pain, feeling tired all time
- Health-related complaints: no time to see the doctor, no time for preventive screenings or vaccinations, teeth are hurting, cold or flu symptoms that linger
- Emotional complaints: feeling anger toward care recipient, feeling guilt about not doing more, feeling depressed, feeling overwhelmed
- Financial complaints: not enough money to take care of loved one, not enough money to take care of household responsibilities
- Indifference about personal hygiene or dress

The Alzheimer's Association (2014) lists many of the complaints above with additional complaints and examples in their 10 signs that a caregiver is stressed:

1. Denial about the disease and its effect on the person who has been diagnosed. *I know Mom is going to get better.*
2. Anger at the person with Alzheimer's, anger that no cure exists or anger that people don't understand what's happening. *If he asks me that one more time I'll scream!*
3. Social withdrawal from friends and activities that once brought pleasure. *I don't care about getting together with the neighbors anymore.*
4. Anxiety about the future. *What happens when he needs more care than I can provide?*
5. Depression that begins to break the spirit and which affects the ability to cope. *I don't care anymore.*
6. Exhaustion that makes it nearly impossible to complete necessary daily tasks. *I'm too tired for this.*
7. Sleeplessness caused by a never-ending list of concerns. *What if she wanders out of the house or falls and hurts herself?*
8. Irritability that leads to moodiness and triggers negative responses and actions. *Leave me alone!*
9. Lack of concentration that makes it difficult to perform familiar tasks. *I was so busy, I forgot we had an appointment.*
10. Health problems that begin to take a mental and physical toll. *I can't remember the last time I felt good.*

Where to Refer

Chapter 8 covers the types of specialists that can become referral sources for caregivers. In general, if there are legal concerns, referrals to legal specialists or to university-run legal clinics may be helpful for matters related to protecting family or patient assets and end-of-life arrangements. Legal professionals such as those specializing in elder care law can also advocate for benefits in behalf of the chronically disabled.

Referrals to social work professionals, agencies like AARP or the local administration on aging, an eldercare specialist, or a geriatric case manager can help with arranging for respite care, in-home care, or nutrition, like Meals on Wheels, and other organizations that provide meals, to help caregivers find some free time to reenergize. Medicare, Medicaid, and private insurance companies will cover some costs of home health care, depending on the services needed. Referrals to Medicare home health care services, Regional Home Health Intermediary, the National Family Caregiver Support Program (through the area Agency on Aging), and Medicaid will help caregivers learn what they are eligible for and how they can pay for home health services.

Making appropriate referrals when caregivers express difficulties with coping is time sensitive. Recognizing changing support needs will enable practitioners to provide more relevant counseling and referrals to appropriate professionals. On a final note, intervention does not end with referrals. Follow-up on referrals and periodic evaluations by the speech-language pathologist or audiologist will be important determinants of positive change in the caregiver's ability to provide care.

Summary

In this chapter, issues of scope of practice and ethical boundaries are discussed to advise speech-language pathologists and audiologists about appropriate education, training, and counseling family caregivers within the clinical setting. From the policy statements generated by the American Speech-Language-Hearing

Association and the American Academy of Audiology, it is clear that practitioners have a role to play in supporting caregivers by:

- providing information on the nature and cause(s) of communication disorders;
- training caregivers in methods for communicating more effectively with the communicative impaired adult;
- being a compassionate listener who builds an environment of trust;
- suggesting or implementing stress-reducing activities;
- organizing information into user-friendly formats for caregivers with low literacy or for whom English is not a primary language;
- beginning discussions about areas of emotional and other needs;
- acknowledging emotions and recommending strategies for alleviating stress;
- directing caregivers to sources of information about issues of concern on a myriad of topics vital to their ability to carry out their caregiving responsibilities;
- recognizing the signs that a caregiver is being overwhelmed by the responsibilities of caregiving;
- making referrals to appropriate professionals when areas of need are outside of the clinical scope of practice in speech-language pathology and audiology;
- respecting cultural traditions and sensitivities when making referrals; and
- engaging in ongoing conversations to determine effectiveness of interventions in education, training, and counseling.

In conclusion, speech-language pathologists and audiologists can do a great deal to lessen the strain and burden often experienced by caregivers. Within the professional toolkits should be sufficient information to educate caregivers about communication or swallowing disorders, training strategies to improve interpersonal communication with an adult with communication or swallowing disorders, a list of resources that address a variety of caregiver concerns, a willingness to engage in sensitive and perceptive listening for when a caregiver needs assistance, and a list of referral sources for those who require intervention from other professionals.

References

Alzheimer's Association. (2014). *Caregiver stress*. Retrieved from https://www.alz.org/care/alzheimers-dementia-caregiver-stress-burnout.asp

American Academy of Audiology (AAA). (2012). *Standards of practice in audiology*. Retrieved from http://audiologyweb.s3.amazonaws.com/migrated/StandardsofPractice.pdf_539978afe9df9182779963.pdf

American Speech-Language-Hearing Association (ASHA). (2004a). *Scope of practice in audiology* [Scope of practice]. Retrieved from http://www.asha.org/policy

American Speech-Language-Hearing Association (ASHA). (2004b). *Preferred practice patterns for the profession of speech-language pathology* [Preferred practice patterns]. Retrieved from http://www.asha.org/policy

American Speech-Language-Hearing Association (ASHA). (2006). *Preferred practice patterns for the profession of audiology* [Preferred practice patterns]. Retrieved from http://www.asha.org/policy

American Speech-Language-Hearing Association (ASHA). (2007). *Scope of practice in speech-language pathology* [Scope of practice]. Retrieved from http://www.asha.org/policy

American Speech-Language-Hearing Association (ASHA). (2008). *Guidelines for audiologists providing informational and adjustment counseling to families of infants and young children with hearing loss birth to 5 years of age* [Guidelines]. Retrieved from http://www.asha.org/policy

American Speech-Language-Hearing Association (ASHA). (2010r). *Code of ethics* [Ethics]. Retrieved from http://www.asha.org/policy

Cameron, J. L., & Cignac, M. A. (2008). "Timing it right": A conceptual framework for addressing the support needs of family caregivers to stroke survivors from the hospital to the home. *Patient Education and Counseling, 70*, 305–314.

Carteret, M. (2011). *Health care for Middle Eastern patients and their families*. Retrieved from http://www.dimensionsofculture.com/2010/10/health-carefor-middle-eastern-patients-families

Carver, C. S. (1997). *Brief COPE*. Retrieved from http://www.psy.miami.edu/faculty/ccarver/index.phtml

DiLollo, A., & Neimeyer, R. A. (2014). *Counseling in speech-language pathology and audiology.* San Diego, CA: Plural.

Flasher, L. V., & Fogle, P. T, (2012). *Counseling skills for speech-language pathologists and audiologists* (2nd ed., pp. 3–37). Clifton Park, NY: Delmar Cengage Learning.

Gallagher-Thompson, D., Tzuang, M., Hinton, L., Alvarez, P., Rengifo, J., Valverde, I., . . . Thompson, L. W. (2015) Effectiveness of a fotonovela for reducing depression and stress in Latino dementia family caregivers. *Alzheimer Disease & Associated Disorders.* Advance online publication. doi:10.1097/WAD.0000000000000077

Harvard Medical School. (2012). *Caregiver's handbook. A Harvard Medical School special health report.* Boston, MA: Harvard Health Publications.

Holland, A. L. (2007). *Counseling in communication disorders: A wellness perspective.* San Diego, CA: Plural.

Holland, A. L., & Nelson, R. L. (2014). *Counseling in communication disorders* (2nd ed.). San Diego, CA: Plural.

Honaker, J. A., & Kretschmer, L. W. (2014). Impact of fear of falling for patients and caregivers: Perceptions before and after participation in vestibular and balance rehabilitation therapy. *American Journal of Audiology, 23,* 20–33.

Jungbauer, J., Döll, K., & Wilz, G. (2008). Gender- and age-specific aspects of assistance needs in caregivers of stroke patients: Results from a qualitative panel study. *Rehabilitation, 47,* 145–149.

Martinez, S. (2008). *Photonovelas in health education. Improving patient outcomes in primary care.* Presentation at the Health Literacy Conference, Howard University Hospital, Washington, DC.

Mason-Baughman, M. B., & Lander, A. (2012). Communication strategy training for caregivers of individuals with dementia. *Perspectives on Gerontology, 17,* 78–83. doi:10.1044/gero17.3.78

McIntyre, C. (2012). *A careful look at the 3 stages of caregiving.* Retrieved from http://www.caringtoday.com/get-basic-caregiving/a-careful-look-at-the-3stages-of-caregiving

Palmer, C. V., Adams, S. W., Bourgeois, M., Durrant, J., & Rossi, M. (1999). Reduction in caregiver-identified problem behaviors in patients with Alzheimer's disease post-hearing-aid fitting. *Journal of Speech, Language, and Hearing Research, 42,* 312–328. doi:10.1044/jslhr.4202.312

Payne, J. C. (2014). *Adult neurogenic disorders: Assessment and treatment. A comprehensive ethnobiological approach* (2nd ed.). San Diego, CA: Plural.

Payne, J. C., & Wright-Harp, W. (2014). Delivering culturally competent services to adults with neurogenic cognitive-language disorders.

In J. C. Payne (Ed.), *Adult neurogenic disorders: Assessment and treatment. A comprehensive ethnobiological approach* (2nd ed., pp. 41–56). San Diego, CA: Plural.

Raina, P., McIntyre, C., Zhu, B., McDowell, I., Santaguida, I., Kristianssen, B., . . . Chambers, L. (2004). Understanding the influence of the complex relationships among informal and formal supports on the well-being of caregivers of persons with dementia. *Canadian Journal on Aging, 23*(Suppl. 1), S49–S59.

Salas-Provance, M. B. (2012). Counseling in a multicultural society: Implications for the field of communication disorders. In L. V. Flasher, & and P. T. Fogel (Eds.), *Counseling skills for speech-language pathologists and audiologists* (2nd ed., pp. 159–184). Clifton Park, NY: Delmar Cengage Learning.

Sörensen, S., Pinquart, M., & Duberstein, P. (2002). How effective are interventions with caregivers? An updated meta-analysis. *Gerontologist, 42*, 356–372.

Tanner, D. C. (2003). *The psychology of neurogenic communication disorders: A primer for health care professionals.* Boston, MA: Allyn & Bacon.

Tanner, D. C. (2008). *The family guide to surviving stroke and communication disorders* (2nd ed.). Boston, MA: Jones & Bartlett.

Thompson, E. H., Futterman, A. M., Gallager-Thompson, D., Rose, J. M., & Lovett, S. B. (1993). Social support and caregiving burden in family caregivers of frail elders. *Journal of Gerontology, 48*, S245–S254. doi:10.1093/geronj/48.5.S245

8

When and Where to Refer Family Caregivers

Wilhelmina Wright-Harp

An integral part of the scope of speech-language pathology and audiology practice involves collaboration with and referral to other professionals (ASHA, 2004, 2005, 2007b). Both are crucial when working with caregivers and their families in service delivery to individuals with severe disabilities resulting from cognitive, communication, and/or swallowing disorders that are neurologically based (e.g., cerebrovascular accident, traumatic brain injury) or due to progressive neurological impairments (e.g., Parkinson's or Alzheimer's disease). As part of a comprehensive approach to interdisciplinary care, it is important to know the expertise of other professionals and their roles to ensure appropriate referrals. Also essential is knowing under what circumstances to refer when the needs of the client/patient and caregiver are out of the speech-language pathologist's scope of practice, thus allowing for best practices in service delivery.

As part of our charge to be clinically and culturally competent (ASHA, 2011; Payne & Wright-Harp, 2014), speech-language pathologists (SLPs) and audiologists (AUDs) must determine when it is necessary to seek the advice of and refer to other professionals. An essential component of this process is knowledge of the roles and responsibilities of all professionals who are service providers to the geriatric population as well as understanding the implications of the impact of caregiving on individuals engaged in ongoing care of a severely ill loved one. It is also important to understand the need for related assessments and procedures that may facilitate thorough patient care. In order to achieve these goals, clinicians must develop the following skills: (a) the ability to identify the roles of other professionals who are service providers for the geriatric population; (b) the ability to apply knowledge to initiate timely and pertinent referrals; (c) the use of appropriate referral procedures; and (d) the ability to collaborate with other professionals in interpreting information and planning culturally appropriate interventions. Understanding the critical nature of how to make effective referrals will not only improve the client's overall quality of care, but also help relieve the caregiver and family of unnecessary stress. Ultimately, the overall long-term outcome will be improved health and wellness of both the client/patient and family (Faison, Faria, & Frank, 1999).

The purpose of this chapter is twofold. First, information will be provided on the network of allied health and other professionals to whom referrals can be made as well as their roles in service delivery to geriatric clients/patients and their families. A second purpose is to address when such referrals are necessary as well as how to effectively communicate and work collaboratively with other service providers to ensure optimum outcomes in service delivery.

Specialists

Specialists who may be appropriate referral sources for caregivers of the geriatric population are attorneys, bereavement coordinators, clinical neuropsychologists, dentists, geriatric care managers, home health case managers, grief counselors, financial advisors, marriage counselors, psychologists, psychiatrists, physicians, neurologists, nurses, physical therapists, occupational therapists, registered dietitians, respiratory therapists, and social workers. In the sections that follow, each profession will be discussed in regard to areas of expertise as well as possible reasons for referrals.

Attorney

The services of an attorney may be required to assist both caregivers and their loved ones with the legal issues that arise related to health care, finances and property. For such matters, it is crucial that the loved one play an integral role in the planning necessary for management of his or her affairs. Such decisions must be finalized before a crisis occurs, while the geriatric individual is capable of making decisions about their welfare. If a large estate is involved, it is advisable that referrals be made to an attorney to provide the necessary legal counsel and assistance with preparation and filing of legal documents such as an Advanced Healthcare Directive, Power of Attorney, and estate planning for disbursement of finances and property (American Bar Association, 2005).

Advance Healthcare Directive

Also known as living will, personal directive, or advanced directive, the Advance Healthcare Directive is a document in which a person specifies what type of medical treatment should or should not be taken for health care in the event that he or she is no longer able to make such decisions due to illness, injury, or incapacity. An attorney is not required for preparation of an advanced health care directive; however, some states require that health care directives be in the form of a legal document. The Advance Healthcare Directive delineates instructions for health care professionals in cases where a person becomes incapacitated and is unable to make decisions for themselves (American Bar Association, 2005; Sitarz, 2002). The health care proxy (i.e., the person chosen to make health care decisions) is known by various names in different states such as health care agent, proxy, representative, attorney-in-fact, surrogate, or even patient advocate. This individual may be the caregiver or another family member or relative but cannot be the health care provider.

Other examples of advanced directives are the Five Wishes and My Directives. The Five Wishes meets the legal requirements in 40 states and addresses the following five areas that are useful in assisting doctors and family in making health decisions and may be ordered from http://www.agingwithdignity.org/catalog/product_info.php?products_id=87 :

1. Who the patient has designated to make the health care decisions when no longer able
2. Medical treatment the patient does and does not want
3. How comfortable the patient wants to be
4. What services and treatments the patient wishes to have
5. What the patient wants loved ones to know

An advanced directive can be created through My Directives online (https://mydirectives.com/).

Power of Attorney (POA)

The POA "is a written authorization to represent or act on another's behalf in private affairs, financial, business, or some other legal matter, sometimes against the wishes of the other. The person authorizing the other to act is the principal, grantor, or donor (of the power). The one authorized to act is the agent or the attorney," (Clifford, 2013).

In instances where the loved one has a progressive illness (e.g., Alzheimer's dementia), a durable power of attorney (DPOA) is an appropriate option. However, the document must be created by the person while he or she has the mental capacity deemed necessary to make such a decision. In the case of a durable power of attorney, the document remains in effect, if the person becomes incapacitated (Clifford, 2013). In instances where the person is incapacitated, and a DPOA does not exist, the only possible option to allow another individual to act on his or her behalf would require a court-imposed conservatorship or guardianship.

Estate Planning

An attorney's services are recommended for preparation of a DPOA, for finances and property, and for management of property and finances. Not only does estate planning help both the caregiver and loved one to have peace of mind, but it also aids in the transition process when the caregiver must assume the primary management of a loved one's affairs. The estate plan allows the loved one to control assets and property while alive and well, establishes a plan of action in the case of disability, and designates the distribution of assets in the preferred manner. The estate would include all assets including home or another property (autos, boats, etc.), bank accounts, stocks, bonds, insurance policies, annuities, IRA, 401(k) plans, to name a few. Also considered part of the estate would be legal documents such as a will (living will), trust, power of attorney (health directive or financial), and designations for beneficiaries of assets.

Bereavement Coordinator

Referrals are made to the bereavement coordinator following the loss of a loved one. The coordinator directs personnel to ensure that the physical, emotional, therapeutic, and spiritual needs of patients and their families are met. Thus, the bereavement coordinator oversees a variety of tasks that may include making funeral or memorial service arrangements, arranging family counseling, and helping the family to follow health care directives stipulated by the patient as part of a living will.

Bereavement coordinators are employed in a variety of medical settings including hospice, nursing homes, hospitals, and home health. Medical speech-language pathologists frequently refer to and work with these specialists. Bereavement coordinators serve as the chief manager overseeing the volunteers, medical staff, health professionals, and others who are involved in helping families during the grieving process. Their role varies depending on the medical setting and particular circumstances of the patient. For example in a hospice facility, the bereavement coordinator initially functions to ensure that the family and the patient are provided optimum care and comfort.

Clinical Neuropsychologist

Clinicians often work collaboratively with clinical neuropsychologists when treating individuals with cognitive-communication disorders (ASHA, 2003). These professionals provide evaluation, diagnostic, treatment, and rehabilitation services to patients across the life span who present with developmental, medical, neurological, and psychiatric conditions (American Board of Professional Psychology, 2014).

A clinical neuropsychologist is consulted when a cognitive assessment and diagnosis is necessary to verify an individual's mental status. In these circumstances, a referral is made to determine whether an individual is capable of making sound decisions regarding their welfare. In the event that the person is diagnosed with a condition such as dementia that makes him or her unable to do so, a family member or caregiver may be recommended to assume adult guardianship. The clinical neuropsychologist's expertise is critical in such cases as the diagnosis is key to determining whether the guardian might be appointed to make decisions about the individual's finances, medical, and personal care.

Clinical neuropsychologists are doctoral-level psychologists who hold a state license to provide diagnostic and intervention services. These specialists utilize psychological, neurological, or physiological methods to evaluate patients' cognitive and emotional strengths and weaknesses and relate these findings to normal and abnormal central nervous system functioning. This information is used in combination with input provided by other medical/health care providers to identify and diagnose neurobehavioral disorders, conduct research, counsel patients and their families, or plan and implement intervention strategies (American Board of Professional Psychology, 2014).

Guidelines for clinical psychologists were established by Division 40, the Clinical Neuropsychology Division of the American Psychological Association (APA), in conjunction with the International Neuropsychological Society (APA, 1989). The National Academy of Neuropsychology (NAN, 2001), which updated these guidelines, defines a clinical neuropsychologist as "a professional within the field of psychology with special expertise in the applied science of brain-behavior relationships. Clinical neuropsychologists use this knowledge in the assessment, diagnosis, treatment, and/or rehabilitation of patients across the lifespan with neurological, medical, neurodevelopmental and psychiatric conditions, as well as other cognitive and learning disorders" (NAN, 2001 p.1).

Clinical neuropsychologists are particularly qualified to formally evaluate emotional states and to provide intervention using applied principles of both experimental and clinical psychology. "Such approaches include, but are not limited to, psychological testing (including objective and projective approaches), personality assessment, behavior analysis, psychotherapy, behavior modification, and group interventions" (ASHA, 2003, p. 9).

Other services provided by clinical neuropsychologists include consultation with other professionals in diverse settings, preventative intervention, research that is clinically relevant, supervision, teaching, and management activities (e.g., program development and administration). As for other disciplines, it is expected that clinical neuropsychologists are both clinically and culturally competent through both knowledge of and sensitivity to culturally diverse populations (Rivera, Byrd, Saez, & Manly, 2010; APA, 1989).

Dentist

Dentists are often professionals to whom referrals are made when issues arise concerning a patient's oral health. When working with dysphagia patients, health care providers make referrals to a dentist to evaluate and treat gingival and dental dysfunction. Dentists may recommend prosthetics to improve swallowing. With advancing age, many elderly clients/patients are at increased risk for a variety of oral health problems (American Dental Association, 2014). See Table 8–1 for a list of common oral conditions frequently observed in the elderly.

Two major reasons to refer to a dentist would be the presence of dental problems that affect oral health leading to weight loss and the long-term effect of periodontal disease on overall health. Dental problems ranging from xerostomia (dry mouth) to periodontal disease frequently occur in aging adults. Moreover, it has been shown that numerous diseases in the body are directly related to poor dental and oral hygiene. In fact, with careful examination of the dentition, gingiva, and tongue, dentists have found evidence of heart or liver disease, eating disorders, diet deficiencies, anemia, diabetes, arthritis, osteoporosis,

Table 8–1. Common Dental Conditions Found in the Geriatric Population

Condition	Etiology
Darkened teeth	Changes in dentin observed in individuals who consume foods and beverages that cause stains (coffee, tea, cocoa, etc.)
Gingivitis	Results from the accumulation of plaque and food debris in the mouth; other causes include the use of tobacco products, poor fitting bridges and dentures, poor diets, and specific diseases including anemia, cancer, and diabetes frequently observed in the geriatric population
Reduced sense of taste	Normal aging process impairs the sense of taste as well as certain diseases, medications, and dentures which can cause sensory loss
Root decay	Caused by prolonged exposure of the tooth root to decay causing acids that can result in cases of gingivitis or periodontal disease
Stomatitis (denture induced)	Results from inflammation of tissue underlying ill-fitting dentures; some causes are ill-fitting dentures, poor dental hygiene, or the accumulation of a fungus (*Candida albicans*) which inflames the gingiva (gums)
Tooth loss	Gingivitis is the major cause of tooth loss in the elderly
Oral thrush	Caused by an overgrowth of the fungus *Candida albicans* in the mouth, a condition that may result when diseases or medications affect the immune system; this form of thrush can develop quickly and if untreated can then turn into a long-lasting chronic infection; symptoms of oral thrush are small white lesions found inside the mouth on the tongue or cheeks; can also be found on the roof of the mouth and gums; below the surface white lesion is a painful, red area that may bleed if the lesion is scraped off
Uneven jawbone	Results from teeth shifting into open spaces following tooth loss; often occurs from failure to replace missing teeth
Xerostomia (dry mouth)	A condition resulting from reduced saliva; may result from radiation treatments for cancers of the head and neck regions; other possible causes are medications (e.g., antihistamines, cold remedies and antidepressants) as well as a condition known as Sjögren's syndrome; numerous medications can cause xerostomia including a common over-the-counter treatment often used by the elderly for toothaches

and autoimmune diseases. Most recently, studies have shown a correlation between dental disease and heart disease. In essence, diminished oral health can affect one's overall health.

One of the most common oral conditions found in the older adults is xerostomia (dry mouth) that often results from the ingestion of multiple medications (polypharmacy). The more medications (both prescription and over the counter) an individual takes, the more likely that xerostomia will result. As a preventative measure, elderly patients should receive regular dental check-ups.

Dentures are more commonly found in the elderly population. However, certain conditions including gingivitis, stomatitis, and reduced oral sensation occur more frequently among the elderly who wear dentures. Good oral health may be difficult to maintain because certain medical conditions, like arthritis affecting the hands and fingers, may make daily brushing or flossing of the teeth difficult to impossible to perform.

Geriatric Care Manager (GCM)

When caring for a disabled older adult becomes overwhelming for the caregiver and family, a GCM is the professional often sought to address a wide range of issues related to the individual's well-being. Geriatric care managers can provide peace of mind to family members who live a distance away from their elderly loved one. As shown in Table 8–2, GCMs can provide an array of services to help patients achieve their long-term care needs, improve their quality of life, and remain independent.

Geriatric care managers are privately hired by caregivers and include nurses, social workers, and licensed therapists. They are licensed in their specialty field but are unique in that they possess specialized training in the area of elder care. Although there is a fee for their services, charges are made on an hourly basis. Services can be used once, during a crisis, or over an extended period when needed to oversee a loved one's well-being.

According to the National Association of Professional Geriatric Care Managers (NAPGCM, 2015), "a geriatric care manager is a health and human services specialist who acts as a guide and advocate for families who are caring for older relatives or dis-

Table 8–2. Services of the Geriatric Care Manager

Service	Description
Care plan development and coordination	Completes care planning assessments to identify problems, eligibility for assistance and service needs; screens, plans, and monitors home health care workers as well as other health and mental health services
Communication	Communicates with family and other professionals to keep them informed of the client's status and any change in needs
Crisis intervention	Provides crisis intervention counseling by referral to a geriatric counselor or psychologists
Federal and state entitlements	Provides information on state and federal entitlements; may put families in contact with local community programs
Financial services	When families have financial challenges, may help manage bill payments or consult with an accountant or the client's power of attorney
Housing	Assists caregivers and families to evaluate and select appropriate and alternative residential options; also facilitates housing transitions
Legal services	Consults with or makes referrals to elder law attorney, who provides expert opinion to courts for determining level of client care
Liaison	Serves as a liaison by communicating with family and other professionals to keep them informed of the client's status and any change in needs
Medical management	Attends doctor appointments; facilitates communication between doctor, client, and family; when appropriate, monitors the individual's compliance to medical orders and doctor's instructions
Safety and security	Monitors the client at home to ensure a safe environment; recommends equipment to add to personal client safety and security; identifies presence of elder abuse or exploitation and institutes necessary safeguards to ensure the client's welfare
Social activities	Helps enrich the client's quality of life by coordinating opportunities for the client to be involved in social, recreational, or cultural activities
Transportation	Makes arrangements for transportation to and from appointments and required services

Source: http://www.mynursingdegree.com/geriatric-care/career-overview.asp

abled adults. The GCM is educated and experienced in any of several fields related to care management, including, but not limited to nursing, gerontology, social work, or psychology, with a specialized focus on issues related to aging and elder care" (NAPGCM, 2015, p. 2).

The GCM determines the geriatric client's needs and in many instances identifies problems of which the caregiver and family are often unaware. A care management plan is developed by the GCM and is designed to enable clients to maintain their independence as well as to address their safety and security concerns. Establishment of a geriatric care management plan, "allows family members to enjoy their elderly loved one without guilt, shame, or feelings of powerlessness that often overwhelm them without such help" (Ruff-King, 2010, p. 1).

Referral to a GCM is critical when families are unable to provide the day-to-day oversight of their loved ones' care, as this professional provides a valuable service by monitoring the patient and communicating back to the family. Although it is ultimately the responsibility of the family to implement any care plan recommended by the GCM, such guidance can help families make more informed decisions that lead to effective actions to ensure quality care and a better life. Ruff-King (2010) commented that the long-term outcome helps reduce worry, stress, and time off of work for family caregivers through a range of services including advocacy, assessment, monitoring, planning, problem solving, education, and family caregiver coaching.

When families live long distances, the specialist most capable of providing invaluable ongoing oversight and monitoring of their loved one's care is the GCM. According to Ruff-King (2010), the services of geriatric care managers are designed to assist in a variety of areas including housing, home care, medical management, communication, social activities, legal services, financial assistance, federal regulations regarding entitlements, and safety and security.

Grief Counselor

Everyone experiences grief or loss at some point in their lives, and the more significant the loss, the more intense is the level of grief. Each individual is different in the way grief is handled.

Some individuals experience a period of withdrawal and helplessness. Others express anger and are then motivated to take action. Regardless of the reaction, the bereaved person requires the support of others. The grief (or bereavement) counselor is the specialist to whom to refer when grieving persons require assistance.

The role of the grief counselor is multifaceted. It may involve working in hospice care with terminally ill patients, serving as a resource in hospice care to the palliative care team and families of the loved one, or helping families handle the loss of a family member following an unforeseen death caused by head injury or a cerebrovascular accident. When working with a terminally ill patient, grief counselors help the individual and the caregiver come to terms with their particular circumstances through communication or therapy. In such cases, grief counselors often work collaboratively with other professionals and counselors (e.g., bereavement coordinators, speech-language-pathologists, and psychologists) to ensure their patients and caregivers are making progress and having their personal needs met. This may include, for example, an analysis of a patient's grief as well as identifying strategies to help the individual cope with their declining mental and physical condition.

In hospice facilities, the grief counselor helps both the caregiver and family cope with the reality of a loved one's progressive decline. This may involve providing information on the progressive stages of the disorder (e.g., AD) as well as providing mechanisms for the family to begin to grieve the changing cognitive and functional state of their loved one.

The most frequent role for which the grief counselor is well equipped is to assist families through the grieving process following the loss of a loved one. In these circumstances, the caregiver and family receive support from the grief counselor who offers advice, compassion, and various strategies to cope with the void created in their lives. Counseling may be provided in either individual or group sessions, depending on the specific needs of the family.

Financial Advisor

As noted in Chapter 2, the demands of caregiving require both a time and financial commitment. Annually, more than 65 million individuals—over 29% of the U.S. population—provide care for a chronically ill, disabled, or aged family member or friend (American Association of Retired Persons, 2010). On average, caregivers spend 20 hours per week in the care of a loved one with two thirds caring for a relative and one third caring for a parent (National Alliance for Caregiving in collaboration with AARP, 2009, p. 4). Estimated caregiver out-of-pocket expenses average $2,400 per year for expenses required to help care recipients (Gibson & Houser 2007). Furthermore, family caregivers can experience loss in wages and other work-related benefits due to changes in work patterns (Gibson & Houser, 2007). This financial investment is equivalent to approximately $375 billion in unpaid services (National Alliance for Caregiving in collaboration with AARP, 2009).

Many caregivers become financially drained as their resources rapidly are diminished by daily caregiving expenses. In addition, caregivers are often faced with handling the finances of their loved one. Under these circumstances, the financial advisor is the individual to whom a referral should be made to assist the caregiver in managing mounting financial obligations. Managing finances can be a challenge for many caregivers (e.g., sorting through insurance options, medical coverage, and bills from service providers can be a formidable task). However, financial advisors can help examine choices and develop an organizational system that a caregiver can use with bills, insurance, and other medical documents (Kramer, 2014). By developing a system to handle the influx of bills and paperwork, the financial advisor can help alleviate the financial burden of caregivers. They also can help caregivers scrutinize the fees of health service providers to prevent excessive charges. Other services may include providing advice on health insurance and long-term care coverage, as well as legal matters (such as a living will or health care directive).

Home Health Case Manager (HHCM)

SLPs and AUDs can play a vital role as team members and team leaders in the home health care setting. Home health care is an area of growing need and has been for the last decade as patients continue to be discharged from hospitals earlier and require ongoing medical care. For those patients who require continued health care services, the HHCM is the individual responsible for overseeing and coordinating the home health team. The top five primary medical diagnoses of home care clients include CVA (63%), CNS diseases (8%), respiratory diseases (5%), head Injury (3%), and other neoplasms (2%) (ASHA, 2007a). The home health care team will vary depending upon the individual's medical and personal care needs. Some professionals on the home health care team include the speech-language pathologist, occupational therapist, physical therapists, social worker, dietitian, nurse, and home health aide.

When a patient's condition changes and other professionals are required to ensure adequate patient care in the home, the HHCM must be contacted. Some of the responsibilities of the HHCM are as follows:

- Assist in coordinating schedules of the service providers to prevent time conflicts.
- Monitor follow-through of health care providers to ensure that the physician's directives are being met.
- Maintain ongoing communication with the family to help coordinate services with the demands of their personal schedules.
- Evaluate the quality of care to ensure that the patient is showing progress and able to get the types of medical and social services necessary to ensure an improved quality of life.

Marital or Marriage Counselor

The day-to-day stressors of caregiving often place tremendous strain on marital relationships (Faison et al., 1999). When a spouse undertakes a caregiving role, there are many changes in the patterns in which the couple relates, making it essential that each spouse acquire new proficiencies and insights (Schumacher, 1995). The impact of the disability or advancing illness on the quality of the marital relationship may be significant. In such instances, a marital counselor is a typically the best resource to help couples resolve issues that can restore and promote healthy marriage relationships.

Marital counselors identify factors that are contributing to the deterioration of a marriage and provide counseling to resolve these issues which may include assistance in dealing with both the emotional stress and physical obligations involved in caring for a person with a disability. Counselors often strive to be proactive in addressing matters that pose potential problems to the marriage. They also assist both partners to adjust to the changed roles and circumstances in their life. In addition, it may be necessary for counselors to examine the caregiving style of both genders to assist them to develop an approach that will protect their emotional state. The added responsibilities of the caregiver may add new complications to the already complex marital relationship affecting both partners.

Qualifications vary by state; however, the minimum requirement is a bachelor's degree in psychology or sociology. Individuals may hold a master's degree in psychology, sociology, or counseling, and a special marriage counseling certificate or training. Additionally, although not a requirement, it is helpful if the individual has been married.

Nurse

Nurses work in a variety of medical settings and in all instances have an essential role as part of the interdisciplinary team. With dysphagia patients, the nurse works to help both patients and caregivers implement and maintain safe swallowing techniques and compensatory strategies during meals and when taking medications. In the home health setting, the home health nurse (HHN) is the primary medical professional charged with the responsibility of relating the patient's condition and progress to the medical team by serving as the liaison between the patient's primary care physician and family. Members of the medical team (i.e., doctors, social workers, and health aides) depend on the HHN to maintain communication with the family. Thus, the HHN has a critical role which includes providing continuous updates, answering questions as they arise, and indicating when additional treatment or services, such as those of an SLP, physical therapist, or occupational therapist are necessary. Consequently, the work of the HHN helps reduce caregiver burden.

To ensure that the patient's needs are being fully addressed, the HHN conducts an assessment of the caregiving environment and develops plans for early intervention to ensure that the patient's care needs are met (Faison et al., 1999). Caregivers must often rely on the services of an HHN, particularly with severely ill patients who require 24-hour care. In these instances, nurses can meaningfully change the course of caregiving for both the caregiver and patient by respecting the role that each has in managing ongoing care. Reinhard, Given, Petloick, and Bemis (2008) note that it is often difficult for an older patient to accept the need for family help following discharge from the hospital because such help compromises independence. Often, nurses can help patients adjust their perception of independence to a context of family care where giving and receiving care should not be equated with a loss of autonomy (Spillman & Pezzin, 2000). In addition, HHNs have been shown to play an instrumental role in helping to bolster care by relieving caregivers of some of the direct care needs of severely ill patients.

The level of training to become an HHN varies. Most have earned a bachelor's degree in nursing; however, this may vary by state and home health agency to include a nursing program certification, or a two-year associate's degree in nursing. HHNs must be licensed by the state(s) in which they practice. An additional requirement is that they must have completed a clinical rotation or internship, preferably in home health care; however, in some cases, training may occur in a variety of medical facilities.

Psychologist

When caregivers are faced with the mounting stress of caring for their loved one and show signs of burnout, SLPS must make appropriate referrals to other professionals who treat stress-related disorders (Payne, 2009). Psychologists are the best suited professionals to whom referrals should be made as they are qualified to assess, diagnose, and treat stress-related disorders. Through the services of a psychologist, caregivers are better able to maintain a positive outlook resulting in improved quality of care to loved ones (Aging Care, 2014).

Caregiving can be mentally and physically demanding. Some of the most frequent psychological problems associated with burnout include depression, emotional problems, stress/distress, and cognitive problems (Brehaut et al., 2004; Douglas & Daly, 2003; Taylor, 2014). According to Zarit (2006), it is estimated that between 40% and 70% of caregivers have clinically significant symptoms of depression, with approximately one fourth to one half of these caregivers meeting the diagnostic criteria for major depression.

There are many signs that a caregiver is in need of a referral. Some of the common warning signs of caregiver burnout include the following:

- Reduced energy level
- Lowered immune system resulting in less resistance to catching colds or flu
- Constant exhaustion even after having adequate sleep
- Neglected personal needs due to lack of time or loss of interest
- No satisfaction from caregiving, even after spending all free time with caregiving
- Difficulty relaxing, even when help is provided
- Impatience or increasing irritability with loved one
- Feelings of hopelessness, helplessness, and being overwhelmed (U.S. Department of Health and Human Services, 2012)

If any of these signs exist, referral of the caregiver to a psychologist is critical.

In addition to the psychological signs associated with long-term caregiving, caregivers also experience inadequate time for sleep, self-care, and other health-related activities (Schulz & Beach, 1999; Schulz, Newsom, Mittelmark, Burton, Hirsch, & Jackson, 1997). In terms of gender, female caregivers are at greater risk than their male counterparts, reporting higher levels of depression and anxiety symptoms and lower levels of subjective well-being, life satisfaction, and physical health than male caregivers (Miller & Cafasso, 1992; Pinquart & Sörensen, 2006; Yee & Schulz, 2000). The devastating consequence of these psychological and physical problems has resulted in an increased mortality (i.e., 63% greater chance of death within 4 years as compared to noncaregivers) (Schulz & Beach, 1999). When these signs and symptoms are observed, the most appropriate referral would be to a psychologist. See Table 8–3 for signs of stress and helpful solutions.

Psychologists provide a variety of services to ensure the mental health of caregivers. According to APA (2010), these include the following:

- Family Caregiver Assessment—evaluation of family caregivers needs, development of a support plan, and making appropriate referrals

Table 8–3. Signs of Caregiver Stress and Tips for Management

Signs of Caregiver Stress		Tips to Reduce Caregiver Stress
Common Signs of Caregiver Stress		*Possible Ways to Reduce Caregiver Stress*
Physical	Headache, muscle aches, sleeping and eating problems, frequent illness	▪ Identify community resources and support
		▪ Obtain information on aging, the elder's condition, and caregiving
Emotional	Guilt, anger, loneliness, depression, and anxiety	▪ Request assistance from family, friends, and community resources
		▪ Practice stress reduction techniques (e.g., exercise, visualization, yoga)
Mental	Forgetfulness, difficulty making decisions, attention wandering	
		▪ Eat well and get rest
		▪ Set realistic goals and expectations—What can and can't you change?
Interpersonal	Withdrawal, blaming, irritability, impatience, and sensitivity to criticism	▪ Look at long-term planning (e.g., health care, financial, legal)
		▪ Set realistic goals and expectations
Spiritual	Feelings of alienation, and loss of hope, purpose, or meaning	▪ Do something nice for yourself (e.g., take a bubble bath, buy a new book, take a walk)
		▪ Acknowledge the sacrifice that you are making out of love

Source: http://www.caregiverresourcecenter.com/the_caregiver.htm#care_giving_stress

- Caregiver Education and Counseling—identifying available resources and making informed decisions regarding care recipient
- Respite Care—temporary relief from the constant responsibility of caring for an elderly individual with special needs, or who might be at risk of abuse or neglect
- Individual and Group Therapy—assisting family caregivers in their management of stress and the often overwhelming responsibility of caregiving and helping caregivers maintain balance between work and family commitments

Psychiatrist

The ongoing stressors associated with caregiving can be further magnified for caregivers coping with persons with mental illness. The process of caring for a loved one with a mental illness is both complex and demanding. If the demands escalate to a point at which the caregiver is unable to cope, referral to a psychiatrist is often necessary. Psychiatrists are physicians who are specifically trained to evaluate, diagnose, and treat individuals with mental disorders. Mental illness can include a variety of conditions including mood and anxiety disorders, personality disorders, and psychotic disorders, like schizophrenia (APA, 2014). Some of the common diagnosed mental conditions of patients frequently seen in the SLP caseload include bipolar disorder, delirium, severe depression, and post-traumatic stress disorder (PTSD).

Psychiatrists who specialize in working with the geriatric population are trained in the field of geriatric psychiatry. According to the American Psychiatric Association (APA, 2014),

> Geriatric psychiatry emphasizes the biological and psychological aspects of normal aging, the psychiatric impact of acute and chronic physical illness, and the biological and psychosocial aspects of the pathology of primary psychiatric disturbances of older age. Geriatric psychiatrists focus on prevention, evaluation, diagnosis and treatment of mental and emotional disorders in the elderly, and improvement of psychiatric care for healthy and ill elderly patients. (p. 1)

An additional reason to refer to a psychiatrist is the need for a consult if a patient is on prescription medications, or to have the psychiatrist monitor the effects of medications over time. Although a few states including Illinois, Louisiana, and New Mexico allow psychologists to write prescriptions (APA, 2014), it is most likely that patients requiring prescriptions would be referred to a psychiatrist.

Unlike psychologists, psychiatrists complete medical school (usually 8 years) and a residency in mental health, typically in the psychiatric department of a hospital. Upon completion of their residency, these physicians are licensed to practice psychiatry. These specialists hold a doctorate degree, either a PhD or PsyD. The latter degree is held by individuals who are interested in clinical psychology which allows them to treat patients. Psychiatrists are increasingly involved in medication management with other mental health providers (e.g., psychologists, geriatric counselors) providing psychotherapy. Consequently, psychiatrists in private practice primarily receive referrals for evaluation, diagnosis, and requests for medication prescriptions to treat psychiatric disorders.

Primary Care Physician (PCP)

The PCP is a critical part of the interdisciplinary team and typically the individual with whom an SLP might consult regarding the medical status of a patient and/or caregiver in need of medical care. The PCP has the responsibility for the provision of continuing and comprehensive medical care to individuals, families, and communities. Depending on the specific provisions of a patient's health insurance, the PCP is often the only professional authorized to make referrals to physician specialists. Some of the most common medical specialists to whom referrals are made include cardiologists, endocrinologists, orthopedic specialists, gastroenterologists, ophthalmologists, nephrologists, neurologists, and urologists (WebMD, 2014). See Table 8–4 for a list of specialists and the most common medical conditions treated in the adult population.

Table 8–4. Medical Specialists for the Geriatric Population

Specialist	Description	Commonly Treated Conditions
Cardiologist	Specializes in diagnosis and treatment of diseases or conditions of the cardiovascular system (the heart and blood vessels)	<ul><li>Aneurysms</li><li>Angina</li><li>Arrhythmia</li><li>Cardiomyopathy</li><li>Carotid artery disease (arteriosclerosis, atherosclerosis)</li><li>Chronic obstructive pulmonary disease (COPD)</li><li>Coronary heart disease</li><li>Congestive heart failure (CHF)</li><li>Heart attack</li><li>Hypertrophic cardiomyopathy (HCM)</li><li>Mitral valve prolapse (MVP)</li><li>Vasospasm</li></ul>
Endocrinologist	Specializes in the diagnosis and treatment of diseases related to the endocrine glands (the thyroid, parathyroid, hypothalamus, testes, ovaries, pituitary, and pancreas). These diseases can often affect other parts of the body.	<ul><li>Menopause</li><li>Diabetes</li><li>Metabolic disorders</li><li>Lack of growth</li><li>Osteoporosis</li><li>Thyroid diseases</li><li>Cancers of the endocrine glands</li><li>Over- or underproduction of hormones</li><li>Cholesterol disorders</li><li>Hypertension</li><li>Infertility</li></ul>

continues

Table 8–4. *continued*

Specialist	Description	Commonly Treated Conditions
Gastro-enterologist	Specializes in the diagnosis, treatment, and management of diseases involving the digestive track, specifically the colon, esophagus, stomach, pancreas, and liver	• Acute renal failure • Hemorrhoids • Colonic neoplasms • Cancer • Polyps • Diverticulosis • Esophageal reflux • Gastritis • Gastroesophageal reflux (GERD) • Hepatitis • Hiatal hernia • Inflammatory bowel diseases • Ulcerative colitis • Crohn's disease (chronic inflammation of digestive or gastrointestinal tract) • Irritable bowel syndrome • Ulcers
Geriatrician (geriatric physician)	Specializes in treating and managing the medical care of elderly patients; often refer to other specialists as needed	• Arthritis • Diabetes • Hypertension • Vascular pathologies (arteriosclerosis, atherosclerosis)
Nephrologist	Specializes in the diagnosis and treatment of kidney diseases	• Acute renal failure • Chronic kidney disease (CKD) • Dialysis • Polycystic kidney disease (PKD) • Kidney stones • Kidney transplantation • High blood pressure • End-stage renal disease (ESRD)

Table 8-4. *continued*

Specialist	Description	Commonly Treated Conditions
Neurologist	Specializes in the diagnosis and treatment of injury and diseases of the nervous system which includes the brain, spinal cord, and cranial and spinal nerves	Neurological disorders resulting from: • Cerebrovascular accidents (hemorrhagic stroke, ischemic stroke) • Head trauma • Hypertension • Seizure disorders, such as epilepsy • Infections of the nervous system (encephalitis, meningitis, or brain abscesses) • Neurodegenerative disorders, such as amyotrophic lateral sclerosis, multiple sclerosis, and Alzheimer's disease • Spinal cord disorders (i.e., inflammatory and autoimmune disorders)
Ophthalmologist	Medical specialist in the surgical care and prevention of eye disease and injury. Ophthalmologists also specialize in diagnosing, prescribing, and treating all defects, injuries, and diseases of the eye. Like optometrists they are also trained to prescribe and fit corrective lenses (eyeglasses and contacts).	• Conjunctivitis • Diabetic retinopathy • Eye cancer • Macular degeneration • Macular holes • Retinal detachment and tears • Retinitis pigmentosa • Retinoblastoma • Retinopathy of prematurity uveitis

continues

Table 8-4. *continued*

Specialist	Description	Commonly Treated Conditions
Optometrist	A primary eye care provider who specializes in, prescribes, and fits corrective lenses. Optometrists diagnose and treat certain eye diseases as well as prescribe medications for treatment of these diseases.	• Conjunctivitis • Macular degeneration • Cataracts • Diabetic retinopathy • Glaucoma • Myopia • Retinitis pigmentosa

Orthopedic specialist	Specializes in treatment of disorders of the musculoskeletal system	• Fractures and broken bones from falls
		• Carpal tunnel
		• Rotator cuff
		• Osteoarthritis
		• Rheumatoid arthritis
		• Other rheumatic diseases including
		  ▫ Gout
		  ▫ Systemic lupus erythematosus (lupus)
		  ▫ Ankylosing spondylitis
		  ▫ Psoriatic arthritis
		  ▫ Reactive arthritis

Podiatrist	Specializes in the diagnosis and treatment of diseases and conditions (e.g., fractures, breaks) of the foot, ankle, and lower leg; also performs surgery and prescribes medications for treatment of disease or injury to the lower extremities	• Arthropathy (diabetic condition also known as Charcot foot) • Psoriatic arthritis • Callus and corns • Fungal infections • Hallux valgus (bunion) • Keratosis palmaris • Onychocryptosis (ingrown toenail • Osteoarthritis

Table 8–4. *continued*

Specialist	Description	Commonly Treated Conditions
Podiatrist *continued*		• Osteomyelitis (due to streptococcus) • Bone disorders (fractures, breaks, osteomyelitis, bone cancer) • Tarsal tunnel syndrome (TTS) • Neuroma • Metarsalgia
Pulmonologist	Specialist involved in diagnosis and treatment of diseases of the upper (nose, pharynx, and throat) and lower respiratory tract (lungs, bronchial tubes) as well as the heart	• Asthma • Emphysema • Tuberculosis • Complicated infections of the chest • Pulmonary complications of AIDS • Injury • Complications of respiratory diagnostic and therapeutic procedures
Rheumatologist	Specializes in diagnosis and treatment of disorders and conditions of the joints, muscles, and bones	• Arthritis (psoriatic, rheumatoid) • Osteoporosis • Autoimmune disorders (scleroderma and lupus)
Urologist	Specializes in treating urinary tract disorders of both genders and reproductive disorders in males	• Cystitis (bladder infection) • Cancer (uterine, prostrate) • Erectile dysfunction • Pyelonephritis (kidney infection) • Urethritis (urinary tract infection)

Physical Therapist (PT)

The PT is a valued member of the team who specializes in evaluating, diagnosing, and treating problems resulting from motor and sensory impairments. Referrals are made to the PT when patients suffer from motor or sensory impairments that reduce mobility and the ability to engage in activities of daily living. In the case of paresis, or reduced range of motion, PTs help patients regain the use of limbs, teach compensatory strategies to reduce the effect of remaining deficits, and establish ongoing exercise programs to help retain newly acquired skills. Referral to a PT is also appropriate when a patient with dysphagia suffers from sensory loss. The PT works to increase sensation by applying selective sensory stimulation (e.g., thermotactile stimulation) to the affected area. Table 8–5 presents a list of interdisciplinary team members who typically work with dysphagia patients.

Occupational Therapist (OT)

Referrals should be made to the occupational therapist (OT) when caregivers need to be trained in specific skills that will promote safety of their loved ones and to assist them in coping with the challenges of caregiving. A referral to an OT is appropriate when the individual patient is experiencing difficulty with daily activities at the level that puts the patient's safety at risk. The OT often works with stroke patients who need to relearn skills necessary for performing self-directed activities such as meal preparation, personal grooming, dressing, and housecleaning. They also can teach individuals how to adapt to driving and provide on-road training. They help patients learn how to perform complex tasks by having them divide the activity into its component parts, practice each part, then combine the components to perform the whole sequence. They also work with other neurologically impaired patients, like those with apraxia, to improve coordination and relearn how to perform planned actions.

Other areas targeted by the OT include helping patients develop compensatory strategies and modify elements in their

Table 8–5. The Roles of Interdisciplinary Dysphagia Team Members (ASHA Practice Portal—Pediatric Dysphagia/Dysphagia Teams)

Team Member	Role
Dentist	Evaluates and treats gingival and dental dysfunction, and may specialize in prosthetics to improve swallowing
Gastroenterologist	Determines any difficulties with the GI tract; performs diagnostic tests related to the esophageal segment of swallowing; places feeding tubes if the patient needs an alternative to oral feeding
Neurologist	Diagnoses and treats neurological causes of swallowing problems
Nurse	Works with the patient and caregivers in implementing and maintaining safe swallowing techniques and compensatory or facilitation strategies during meals and when taking medications
Nutritionist/ dietician	Evaluates nutritional needs; follows therapy recommendations regarding consistencies of liquids and solid foods; determines needs for special diets; and ensures adequate nutrition when using alternative means of nutrition
Occupational therapist	Evaluates and treats sensory and motor impairments and assesses prosthetic needs related to self-feeding and swallowing
Otolaryngologist	Diagnoses and treats oral, pharyngeal, laryngeal, and tracheal pathologies that may cause or contribute to swallowing problems; cooperates with speech-language pathologist in performing endoscopic evaluations of swallowing (FEES®)
Physiatrist	May coordinate the rehabilitation team during the patient's recovery from acute illness and may follow those with chronic diseases associated with dysphagia on an ongoing basis
Physical therapist	Evaluates and treats body positioning, sensory and motor movements necessary for safe and efficient swallowing, recommends appropriate seating equipment needed during feeding

continues

Table 8–5. *continued*

Team Member	Role
Psychologist	Evaluates and treats patients and their families in adjusting to dysphagia disability, in coping with ramifications of swallowing disorders, and in managing associated stresses; participates on teams treating children with behavioral feeding disorders
Pulmonologist	Evaluates and treats respiratory complications of patients with dysphagia; manages chronic pulmonary diseases and patients/students who are ventilator dependent
Radiation oncologist	Implements radiation therapy protocols to treat patients with cancers of the mouth, throat, and/ or esophagus which may cause dysphagia
Radiologist	Evaluates swallowing problems through radiologic studies, primarily with speech-language pathologists during videofluorographic swallow studies (VFSSs)
Social worker	Assists and counsels patients and families in adjustment to disability, accesses the least-restrictive residential and treatment environments, and deals with third-party payment issues
Speech-language pathologist	Evaluates and treats patients with swallowing problems, including direct modifications of physiologic responses and indirect approaches such as diet modification

Source: American Speech-Language-Hearing Association. (n.d.). *Dysphagia Teams*. Retrieved from http://www.asha.org/Practice-Portal/Clinical-Topics/Pediatric-Dysphagia/Dysphagia-Teams

environments which impact their ability to perform activities of daily living. Patients with hemiparesis involving an arm and hand are taught to substitute Velcro fasteners for buttons on clothing. The OT can also help with home modification to eliminate barriers and increase safety. Examples are the installation of rails on stairs and bars in bathrooms, particularly in the shower.

Nutritionist/Dietitian

In the delivery of services to patients with dysphagia or diabetes, SLPs work collaboratively with the nutritionist/dietician. The dietician evaluates the patient's nutritional needs, follows therapy recommendations regarding food consistencies of liquids and solids, determines needs for special diets, and ensures adequate nutrition when using alternative means of nutrition. The registered dietitian (RD) is a professional trained in nutrition who is typically consulted when there are concerns about patient nutrition. The RD makes diet modifications to ensure the patient has a diet that will provide ample nutrition and caloric intake in cases where patients are experiencing weight loss. These professionals work in hospitals, physician offices, managed care organizations, home health care, and other medical settings.

When working with patients with dysphagia, the SLP determines the appropriate food consistencies to prevent aspiration risk; however, referrals are made to the dietician to ensure that the patient's diet has adequate nutrition. The dietician helps patients determine their food needs based on desired weight, lifestyle, medications, and other health goals (e.g., in patients with diabetes a common goal is lowering fat intake).

Registered Respiratory Therapist (RRT)

The RRT is involved in the assessment, diagnosis, and treatment of respiratory dysfunction. Respiratory therapists apply scientific knowledge and theory to practical clinical problems of respiratory care. The respiratory therapist is qualified to assume primary responsibility for all respiratory care modalities, including the supervision of certified respiratory therapist (CRT) functions. The respiratory therapist may be required to exercise considerable independent clinical judgment, under the supervision of a physician, in the treatment of patients with respiratory dysfunction.

Social Workers

When caregivers require assistance with solving and coping with problems in their lives, referrals are made to a social worker. One subspecialty is that of clinical social worker who diagnoses and treats mental, behavioral, and emotional issues (U.S. Bureau of Labor Statistics, 2014). Social workers may be employed in a variety of settings. Those who work in medical settings have several roles that may include assisting and counseling patients and families to help them adjust to the changes resulting from disability, facilitating patients' access to the least restrictive residential and treatment environments, and working with employers or unions to resolve third-party payment matters (ASHA, 2014).

In a long-term care (LTC) facility, the social worker helps newly admitted patients make the transition from their previous living environment to life in an institutional setting while also meeting the social/emotional comfort needs of those residents. Once patients have transitioned into the LTC facility, the social worker's responsibility is to assure the patients' continuing needs are met and that the patients are given the opportunity to participate in planning for continued care in the facility, transfer, or discharge back into the community. In addition to working with the patients, a considerable amount of the social worker's time may involve working with the families (Perrin & Polowy, 2008).

Summary

There are a number of professionals who can address concerns or issues outside of the scope of practice for speech-language pathologists and audiologists. Caregivers can be referred to some specialists, like the GCM, psychologist, psychiatrist, grief/bereavement and marital/marriage counselors, and specialists who provide in-home health services, to assist them in reducing stress and burden. Other specialists, like the OT, PT, and nutritionist/dietician can assist patients and caregivers or advocate for patient and caregiver services within their areas of expertise. A list of resources for referrals is provided below.

Resources

American Association of Geriatric Psychiatry
http://www.aagponline.org

Administration on Aging (2004), *National Family Caregiver Support Program (FCSP) Complete Resource Guide*
Washington, DC: Author.

Advance Healthcare Directive
https://www.legalnature.com/lp/ahcd/Advanced-healthcare directive?utm_source=Bing&utm_medium=ppc&utm_term=Advance%20Healthcare%20Directive&utm_campaign=Advance +Healthcare+Directive+Form+-+Bing&fid=2744478

American Academy of Clinical Neuropsychology
http://www.theaacn.org

American Speech-Language-Hearing Association
http://www.asha.org

Butts, D. M. (2005). *Kinship Care: Supporting Those Who Raise our Children*
Baltimore, MD: Annie E. Casey Foundation. Retrieved from http://www.aecf.org/initiatives/mc/readingroom/documents/ Kincare.pdf

The Caregiver Resource Center
http://www.caregiverresourcecenter.com/counseling_ services.htm

Commonwealth Fund (2005)
Issue Brief: A Look at Working-Age Caregivers' Roles, Health Concerns, and Need for Support.
Retrieved from http://www.commonwealthfund.org

Easter Seals & the National Alliance for Caregiving (2007). *Caregiving in Rural America*
Retrieved from http://www.easterseals.com

Family Caregiver Alliance (2001). *Selected Caregiver Statistics* **(Fact Sheet)**
San Francisco, CA: Author.

The Five Wishes
Information on Five Wishes:
http://www.agingwithdignity.org/five-wishes.php

List of states that authorize use:
http://www.agingwithdignity.org/five-wishes-states.php

MyDirectives
https://mydirectives.com

National Alliance for Caregiving
http://www.caregiving.org

National Alliance on Mental Illness, Family-to-Family Program
http://www.nami.org

National Association of Professional Geriatric Care Managers
http://www.caremanager.org

National Center on Elder Abuse (NCEA) (2002). Preventing Elder Abuse by Caregivers, Institute on Aging (formerly Goldman Institute on Aging)
Washington, DC

National Family Caregivers Association
http://www.thefamilycaregiver.org

National Stroke Association Caregiving Community (network for caregivers and family of stroke survivors)
http://www.stroke.org/site/PageServer?pagename=sem_care living&gclid=CjwKEAjwj4ugBRD1x4ST9YHplzMSJACTDms8 38WsXppmwFwwDyhwY3ir-YfBRLxKxzm6MjohvY8ZWxoCL 1Lw_wcB

National Alliance for Caregiving in collaboration with AARP (2009). *Caregiving in the United States*
Retrieved from http://www.caregiving.org/data/Caregiving_in_ the_US_2009_full_report.pdf

National Alliance for Caregiving (2004). *Caregiving in the United States*
Washington, DC: Author.

National Alliance for Caregiving (2005). *Young Caregivers in the United States*
Retrieved from
http://www.caregiving.org/data/youngcaregivers.pdf

National Gay and Lesbian Task Force Policy Institute (2005). *Selling Us Short: How Social Security Privatization Will Affect Lesbian, Gay, Bisexual, and Transgender*
Retrieved from http://thetaskforce.org/downloads/reports/reports/SellingUsShort.pdf

Opinion Research Corporation (2005). *Attitudes and Beliefs About Caregiving in the United States: Findings of a National Opinion Survey*
Opinion Research Corporation.

Parents with Disabilities Online (2010)
Retrieved from http://www.disabledparents.net

U.S. Census Bureau (2006). *2005 American Community Survey: Tables S1001 and S1002*
Washington, DC: Author.

References

AgingCare.com. (2014). *The importance of counseling for caregiver burnout.* Retrieved from http://www.agingcare.com/Articles/counseling-for-caregiver-burnout-126208.htm

American Association of Retired Persons. (2010). *Almost one-third of U.S. adult population plays caregiver role in households across America: 65.7 million caregivers.* Retrieved from http://www.aarp.org/about-aarp/press-center/info-032010/caregiving_survey_release.html

American Bar Association. (2005). *Consumer's tool kit for health care advance planning.* Washington, DC: ABA Commission on Law and Aging.

American Board of Professional Psychology. (2014). *Definition of a clinical neuropsychologist.* Retrieved from http://www.abpp.org/i4a/pages/index.cfm?pageid=3304

American Dental Association. (2014). *Elderly: Geriatric population.* Retrieved from http://www.ada.org/en/member-center/oral-health-topics/elderly-care-see-geriatrics

American Psychological Association (APA) Division 40. (1989). Definition of a clinical neuropsychologist. *Clinical Neuropsychologist, 3*(1), 22.

American Psychological Association (APA). (2010). *Presidential Task Force on Caregivers.* Retrieved from http://www.apa.org/about/gr/issues/cyf/caregiving-facts.aspx

American Psychological Association (APA). (2014). *Geriatric psychiatry.* Retrieved from http://www.psychiatry.org/practice/professional-interests/geriatric-psychiatry

American Speech-Language-Hearing Association. (n.d.) *Dysphagia Teams.* Retrieved from http://www.asha.org/Practice-Portal/Clinical-Topics/Pediatric-Dysphagia/Dysphagia-Teams

American Speech-Language-Hearing Association. (2003). *Evaluating and treating communication and cognitive disorders: approaches to referral and collaboration for speech language pathology and clinical neuropsychology* [Technical Report]. Retrieved from http://www.asha.org/policy

American Speech-Language-Hearing Association. (2004). *Knowledge and skills needed by speech-language pathologists and audiologists to provide culturally and linguistically appropriate services* [Knowledge and skills]. Retrieved from http://www.asha.org/policy

American Speech-Language-Hearing Association. (2005). *Evidence-based practice in communication disorders* [Position statement]. Available from http://www.asha.org/policy

American Speech-Language-Hearing Association. (2007a). *ASHA SLP health care survey: Caseload characteristics.* Rockville, MD: Author.

American Speech-Language-Hearing Association. (2007b). *Scope of practice in speech-language pathology* [Scope of Practice]. Retrieved from http://www.asha.org/policy

American Speech-Language-Hearing Association. (2011). *Cultural competence in professional service delivery* [Position statement]. Retrieved from http://www.asha.org/policy

Bureau of Labor Statistics. (2014). *Occupational outlook handbook.* Retrieved from http://www.bls.gov/ooh/community-and-socialservice/social-workers.htm

Brehaut, J. C., Kohen, D. E., Raina, P., Walter, S. D., Russell, D. J., & Rosenbaum, P. (2004). The health of primary caregivers of children with cerebral palsy: How does it compare with that of other Canadian caregivers? *Pediatrics, 114,* e182–e191. doi:10.1542

Caregiver Action Network. (n.d.) *Family caregiver toolbox.* Retrieved from http://www.caregiveraction.org/resources/toolbox/

Clifford, D. (2013). *Making your own living trust* (11th ed.). Berkeley, CA: NOLO.

Douglas, S. L., & Daly, B. J. (2003). Caregivers of long term ventilator patients: Physical and psychological outcomes. *Chest, 123,* 1073–1081. doi:10.1378/chest.123.4.1073

Faison, K. J., Faria, S. H., & Frank, D. (1999). Caregivers of chronically ill elderly persons. *Journal of Community Health Nursing, 16,* 243–253.

Gibson, M., & Houser, A. (2007). *Valuing the invaluable: A new look at the economic value of family caregiving.* Washington, DC: AARP.

Kramer, L. (2014). *Five things to ask before hiring a financial advisor.* Retrieved from http://www.investopedia.com/articles/investing/073114/5-questions-ask-hiring financialadvisor.asp

Miller, B., & Cafasso, L. (1992). Gender differences in caregiving: Fact or artifact? *The Gerontologist, 32,* 498–507.

National Academy of Neuropsychology (NAN). (2001). *Definition of a clinical neuropsychologist.* Retrieved from http://www.nanonline.org/NAN/files/PAIC/PDFs/NANPositionDefNeuro.pdf

National Alliance for Caregiving in collaboration with AARP. (2009). *Caregiving in the U.S.* Retrieved from http://www.caregiving.org/data/Caregiving_in_the_US_2009_full_report.pdf

National Association of Professional Geriatric Care Managers (NAPGCM). (2015). *What you need to know.* Retrieved from http://www.caremanager.org/what-you-should-know/#section2

Payne, J. C. (2009, March 3). Supporting family caregivers: The role of speech-language pathologists and audiologists. *The ASHA Leader.*

Payne, J. C., & Wright-Harp, W. (2014). Delivering culturally competent services to adults with neurogenic cognitive-language disorders. In J. C. Payne (Ed.), *Adult neurogenic language disorders: Assessment and treatment: A comprehensive ethnobiological approach* (2nd ed., pp. 41–56). San Diego, CA: Plural.

Perrin, N., & Polowy, J. (2008). *The role of the social worker in the long-term care facility. Missouri Long-Term Care Ombusman Program.* Retrieved from http://health.mo.gov/seniors/ombudsman/pdf/RoleLTCsocialworker.pdf

Pinquart, M., & Sörensen, S. (2006). Helping caregivers of persons with dementia: Which interventions work and how large are their effects? *International Psychogeriatrics, 18,* 577–595. doi:10.1017/S1041610206003462

Reinhard, S. C., Given, B., Petlick, N. H., & Bemis, A. (2008). Supporting family caregivers in providing care. In R. G. Hughes (Ed.), *Patient safety and quality: An evidence-based handbook for nurses* (Chap. 14).

Rockville, MD: Agency for Healthcare Research and Quality. Retrieved from http://www.ncbi.nlm.nih.gov/books/NBK2665/

Rivera Mindt, M., Byrd, D., Saez, P., & Manly, J. (2010). Increasing culturally competent neuropsychological services for ethnic minority populations: A call to action. *The Clinical Neuropsychologist, 24*(3), 429–453.

Ruff-King, M. (2010). *Geriatric case manager—How geriatric care management can benefit the elderly and their families. Home and family: Elder care.* Retrieved from http://ezinearticles.com/?Geriatric-Case-Manager---How-Geriatric-Care-ManagementCan-Benefit-the-Elderly-and-Their-Families&id=4820252

Schulz, R., & Beach, S. R. (1999). Caregiving as a risk factor for mortality: The caregiver health effects study. *Journal of the American Medical Association, 15*, 2215–2219.

Schulz, R., Newsom, J., Mittelmark, M., Burton, L., Hirsch, C., & Jackson, S. (1997). Health effects of caregiving: The Caregiver Health Effects Study: An ancillary study of the cardiovascular health study. *Annals of Behavioral Medicine, 19*, 110–116.

Schumacher, K. L. (1995). Family caregiver role acquisition: Role-making through situated interactions. *Scholarly Inquiry for Nursing Practices: An International Journal, 9*, 211–226.

Sitarz, D. (2002). *Living wills simplified: Prepare a complete advance health care directive.* Carbondale, IL: Nova.

Spillman, B. C., & Pezzin L. E. (2000). Potential and active family caregivers: Changing networks and the "sandwich generation." *Milbank Quarterly, 78*, 347–374

Taylor, W. D. (2014). Depression in the elderly. *New England Journal of Medicine, 371*, 1228–1236.

U.S. Department of Health and Human Services. (2012) *Caregiver stress fact sheet.* Retrieved from http://womenshealth.gov/publications/ourpublications/fact-sheet/caregiver-stress.html#d

WebMD. (2014). *Types of medical specialists.* Retrieved from http://www.webmd.com/a-to-zguides/medical-specialists-medical-specialists

Yee, J. L., & Schulz, R. (2000). Gender differences in psychiatric morbidity among family caregivers: A review and analysis. *Gerontologist, 40*, 147–164.

Zarit, S. (2006). Assessment of family caregivers: A research perspective. In Family Caregiver Alliance (Eds.), *Caregiver assessment: Voices and views from the field.* Report from a National Consensus Development Conference (Vol. II, pp. 12–37). San Francisco, CA: Family Caregiver Alliance.

9

Epilogue: Case Study

Joan C. Payne

Information given in the previous chapters has shown how speech-language pathologists and audiologists can play important roles in supporting family caregivers of adults with disorders of communication and/or swallowing. In this chapter, a case study is provided that describes both the changing needs of an adult patient with deteriorating chronic conditions and those of the spousal family caregiver. At the end of the case study, a series of questions are included that will allow clinicians to consider possible ways in which to be attuned to areas of educational and counseling needs as well as to the dynamic issues of caregiver stress. These thinking questions are also designed to assist clinicians about when to provide appropriate caregiver information and referrals to outside resources.

This book has been devoted to supporting caregivers because they are the nexus between the health care system and quality of life for persons before and after acute care. In this regard, the focus has been on positive support through providing caregivers with the necessary information, resources, and referrals to enable them to continue their caregiving responsibilities without undue interruptions. Positive support intervention may be seen in Holland and Ryan's (2014) approach to counseling from a wellness perspective. This approach has its roots in positive psychology which is designed to "increase resilience and optimism" in persons who are striving to overcome disasters or catastrophes (Holland & Ryan, 2014). Much of this positive psychology involves educating patients and their families, but other major aspects of counseling also involve listening, giving information, enabling individuals to clarify what they are feeling and thinking, and finally, providing options for changing behaviors.

Counseling to effect change in problem solving can be difficult, particularly if a caregiver resists seeking external support because of cultural mores or traditions. Another perspective is what DiLollo and Neimeyer (2014) called the constructionist theory of counseling that is rooted in contemporary research. In this theory, the counselor intervenes in how a person constructs or interprets meaning of life experiences, both personal and in the interactions with others. Intervention is designed to help the individual, in this case the caregiver, to "understand problematic experiences . . . to launch new and more effective ones" (DiLollo & Neimeyer, 2014, p. 61).

These principles that are recommended as effective strategies for the person with communication or swallowing impairments may also apply to persons who are providing care. In other words, in patient-centered intervention, a systematic approach to supporting caregivers should be an integral part of the clinician's plan for intervention in the communication or swallowing disorder. Many caregivers need the same level of systematic, strategic, and planned support as those for whom they are giving care, as can be seen in the following case study.

Case Study: Mr. and Mrs. F. M.

Mr. F. M. was a 70-year-old man who lived independently in his home. He drove an automobile, was an active participant in his church and community, and even made golf clubs for sale to other golf enthusiasts. A widower for many years, he began to date again in his late sixties. Through mutual friends, he met a woman who was 15 years his junior. After two years of dating, he and his lady friend established an exclusive, loving relationship. They became engaged and set a wedding date. Three months before the wedding, Mr. F. M.'s fiancée rented her house and moved in with Mr. F. M.

Two months before the wedding, Mr. F. M. suffered an ischemic anterior stroke in the left hemisphere and was rushed to the hospital. Speech-language pathology assessment results indicated that his stroke caused a moderate Broca's aphasia with word-finding difficulty and right-side hemiplegia. He was considered to be a promising candidate for speech-language therapy and was scheduled for outpatient therapy twice weekly at the hospital after discharge from acute care.

During his hospitalization, Mr. F. M.'s fiancée, Ms. J. S., expressed concern to his speech-language pathologist of record that she and Mr. F. M. had not yet married and that his family was causing her considerable distress about his property should he become unable to care for himself. According to Ms. J. S., the family had begun to visit their home while her fiancé was in the hospital and to remark that Mr. F. M.'s current will made his brother the sole heir and executor of his estate. In the event of his death, Mr. F. M.'s family stood to inherit everything, including his home. Mr. F. M. had not had an opportunity to make a new will at this point that included his fiancée, and he had not completed paperwork for his fiancée to undertake financial arrangements or make health decisions for him. Under these circumstances, Ms. J. S. was both frightened at the possibility of being displaced from their home and unsure of whether she wanted to take on the tremendous responsibility of caregiving as a spouse.

Subsequently, Mr. F. M. and Ms. J. S. decided to marry within a month after his discharge from the hospital. The now-Mrs. F. M. was still working, and she returned to work full time. Mr. F. M. attempted to clean the house and prepare dinner for his wife, but was often forgetful about his chores and unable to complete them without error. Although his wife left simple, written instructions for him for his daily chores, he had difficulty with reading and writing with his dominant hand.

Coming home to burned dinners and a disordered house after working all day caused his wife considerable distress. Other problems were that there were fewer and fewer occasions of intimacy, and that Mr. F. M. had to be readmitted to the hospital on five different occasions to have carotid stents put in place.

After each stent procedure, Mr. F. M. appeared to be less cognitively engaged and less talkative. Mrs. F. M. began to complain that she had no one to talk to in the evenings after work. Most evenings, while Mr. F. M. sat in the dining room alone, Mrs. F. M. talked about his medical crises with friends on the telephone.

Mr. F. M. began to miss appointments for speech-language therapy and audiological assessments because he had no one to bring him to the hospital's outpatient clinic. Also, his insurance would run out periodically for rehabilitation services. When his insurance was viable for speech-language pathology and audiological services, his wife worked all day and was unable to get away to pick him up or take him home. Sitting alone in his home all day did little to encourage him to communicate. His expressive language deteriorated further, and there were signs of cognitive impairment in attention, comprehension, memory, and focus. Mrs. F. M. grew increasingly impatient with her husband and with his family who offered no assistance to her for his care. Mr. F. M.'s physical condition also deteriorated. He had bouts of bowel and bladder incontinence and had a number of "accidents" at night that Mrs. F. M. had to clean up before going to work. Increasingly, he needed help with ambulation and his personal hygiene.

Mr. F. M.'s personality began to change. Prior to his stroke, he had been an affable, positive, and kindly person. As his language and cognitive skills declined, he was becoming frustrated with his inability to communicate with his wife and was, on occasion, hostile and sometimes verbally abusive toward her. Mrs. F. M. became more and more intolerant of his verbal outbursts and continued to talk about him within his earshot on the telephone with her friends. When she was able to bring him to outpatient rehabilitation, Mrs. F. M. complained to the speech-language pathologist that she needed a vacation from the day-to-day work of caring for her husband. She reported being tired all the time and that the stress of his care was impinging on her relationships at work. She had begun to receive poor evaluations for job performance and felt that her position of over 25 years was in jeopardy.

This case study does not have a happy ending. Toward the end of her husband's life, Mrs. F. M. gave every indication that she was extremely stressed by her husband's condition and told his speech-language pathologist that he had attempted to hit her when he could not make himself understood. She also related that she hit him back in retaliation. The day after sharing this information, Mrs. F. M. found her husband dead at home of an apparent heart attack. In addition to her grieving and feelings of guilt, Mrs. F. M. expressed intense feelings that her husband's family did not offer to assist her with making the final funeral arrangements. During the following year, Mrs. F. M.'s own health deteriorated. She experienced a number of health problems, including a blood clot in her leg which she ignored. Within the year, she, too, was found dead at home.

Commentary

Mr. F. M. was the focus of therapy for his aphasia and word-finding impairment, but his caregiver also needed a program of planned support as well. It is not uncommon for persons who become caregivers to find themselves adrift when it is their turn to assume full responsibility for giving care. Much of what this case presentation shows is a spousal caregiver who is stunned to find that her dreams for a new and successful marriage are thwarted by a catastrophic illness that changes the entire landscape of her views about her new husband, her role as a wife, and their future together. From her expressed concerns, she was repeatedly overwhelmed by her husband's functional limitations (Blake, Lincoln, & Clarke, 2003), changes in intimacy between them (Thompson & Ryan, 2009), the progressive nature of his chronic disabilities, and by his behavioral changes (Thompson & Ryan, 2008).

Some research has shown that women, whether stroke survivors or caregivers for persons with aphasia after stroke, tend to accept responsibility for continuing their prestroke roles. By contrast, male stroke survivors relinquish some of their roles, transferring the responsibilities onto their spouses (Blake et al., 2003). Mrs. F. M. had moved away from her family to find better opportunities for employment, had very limited outside support from her husband's family, and relied heavily on her network of friends to help her to cope. Although she accepted many of the prestroke responsibilities of marriage, she was in need of considerable external support to remain healthy and confident that she could do an effective job of caregiving.

The clinicians for Mr. F. M. often made time for his wife to discuss her concerns and to help her with solving problems in the home as they arose. It would have been most helpful and perhaps less time intensive if Mr. F. M.'s clinicians had an available toolkit of information that addressed caregiver concerns. Such a toolkit could include, for example, a listing of local agencies and institutions that provide free transportation to health care services. Similarly, a list of names and costs for area home health services such as certified nurses' aides, hired companions and homemakers, and home health aides, may have relieved a great deal of stress about meal preparation and light housekeeping, and most importantly, companionship. Descriptions of types, costs, and locations of assistive devices (or augmentative devices) may have improved some areas of Mr. F. M.'s communication and decreased the couples' frustration significantly. Mrs. F. M.'s feelings of depression, grief, anger, and helplessness in the face of her husband's steady and progressive changes in health and communication may have been alleviated by referrals to grief or pastoral counselors and to psychologists and psychiatrists.

This case study may have turned out differently if the caregiver had been provided with strategic areas of resource information and a planned program of intervention. Planning should have included counseling and education that was appropriate for her husband's changing health status, and routine referrals to professionals who could have alleviated her concerns for her and her husband's future.

Think Questions

Clinicians are often faced with very real-life problems as they listen to caregivers. The reader is referred to Chapter 7 for a listing of websites for caregivers and to Chapter 8 for descriptions of other professionals' responsibilities as these relate to caregiver issues. The following questions are posed to help speech-language pathology and audiology clinicians provide assistance to caregivers in their intervention plans:

1. What resources could the clinician have provided to Mrs. F. M. to help her with the legal issues of will preparation, power of attorney, and advance directives? Which resources would have helped both partners with issues of financial literacy?
2. What information could the clinician have shared with Mrs. F. M. about laws affecting her job status as a caregiver?
3. What strategies could the clinician have shared with Mrs. F. M. to help with getting her husband to and from his medical or rehabilitation appointments?
4. What could the clinician have recommended as assistive devices (or augmentative devices in the case of a hearing-impaired adult) to address Mr. F. M.'s decreasing ability to make himself understood?
5. Were there home services that the clinician could have advised Mrs. F. M. about for help with her husband's personal hygiene, meal preparation, and housekeeping? Which ones?
6. What referrals would have been appropriate to recommend for Mrs. F. M. to assist her with
   a. respite from the intensive work of caregiving;
   b. coping with the grief from seeing her new marriage and new husband deteriorate;
   c. managing stressors related to her relationship with her husband's family;
   d. physical self-care;
   e. marital counseling;
   f. spiritual support; and
   g. end-of-life care.
7. With reference to Question 6, what culturally sensitive considerations should be included in making referrals for persons from diverse ethnic, cultural, or religious backgrounds?
8. In what ways could the clinician have helped to educate Mrs. F. M. about the effects of stents and repeated hospitalizations on her husband's cognitive status?
9. If cognitive changes were documented during periodic assessment, how could the clinician have helped Mrs. F. M.

to change her husband's environment to give him more opportunities to use his residual communication or cognitive skills (e.g. senior day care, communication partners, to name a few)?

10. What could the clinician have suggested to Mrs. F. M., to help her find a community of persons also coping with aphasia and dementia (e.g., support groups, websites, and associations in addition to her telephone friends)?

11. Several assessments are commonly used by health professionals to measure caregiver strain. Referring to Chapter 7, are there assessments that speech-language pathologists or audiologists could have used to begin the discussions about Mrs. F. M.'s needs for education, counseling, or referrals?

Summary

Adults with acute and chronic conditions are living longer and will continue to need help from family and friends. This case study is not uncommon among caregivers who are often quite different from those of the previous generation. Many caregivers are presently managing caregiving long-distance or are living far from the communities of their childhood where they may have had more of an extensive family support network to assist them while they are providing care. Although dependent on assistance from a caregiver, some persons with communication or swallowing impairments may be divorced or widowed and find themselves either alone or in new marriages and relationships that have not stood the test of time. The stress of caregiving in a relatively new relationship may be particularly overwhelming for both the person with disabilities and the caregiver.

One way to address caregiver stress is to define early what problems may arise. Developing a plan of action for and with caregivers is highly recommended in the *Caregiver's Handbook* published by Harvard Medical School as a Special Health Report (2012). Included in the Harvard plan is a needs questionnaire that caregivers can complete with their loved one and the speech-language pathologist or audiologist to stimulate ideas and eliminate possible causes of conflict that can cause breakdowns in communication. It is important for a caregiver and a care recipient to set goals, identify areas that are problematic, and find possible solutions. It is also important that caregivers and the persons receiving care have regularly scheduled opportunities with their clinician to review their goals and problem areas since change is inevitable in caregiving. Speech-language pathologists and audiologists have, by virtue of training and focus on human behavior, unique opportunities to make a difference in the quality of life of persons who are caring for adults with disorders of communication or swallowing.

References

Blake, H., Lincoln, N. B., & Clarke, D. D. (2003). Caregiver strain in spouses of stroke patients. *Clinical Rehabilitation, 17*, 312–317.

DiLollo, A., & Niemeyer, R. A. (2014). *Counseling in speech-language pathology and audiology: Reconstructing personal narratives* (pp. 51–71). San Diego, CA: Plural.

Harvard Medical School Special Health Report. (2012). *Caregiver's handbook*. Boston, MA: Harvard Health Publications.

Holland, A. L., & Ryan, R. L. (2014). *Counseling in communication disorders: A wellness perspective* (2nd ed., pp. 1–58). San Diego, CA: Plural.

Thompson, H. S., & Ryan, A. (2008). A review of the psychosocial consequences of stroke and their impact on spousal relationships. *British Journal of Neuroscience Nursing, 4*, 177–184.

Thompson, H. S., & Ryan, A. (2009). The impact of stroke consequences on spousal relationships from the perspective of the person with stroke. *Journal of Clinical Nursing, 18*, 1803–1811. doi:10.1111/j.1365-2702.2008.02694.x

APPENDIX A

Guidelines for Audiologists Providing Informational and Adjustment Counseling to Families of Infants and Young Children With Hearing Loss Birth to 5 Years of Age*

About This Document

This guidelines document is an official statement of the American Speech-Language-Hearing Association (ASHA). The ASHA Scope of Practice in Audiology states that the practice of audiology includes providing services to individuals across the entire age span from birth through adulthood. The Guidelines for the

*American Speech-Language-Hearing Association. (2008). Guidelines for audiologists providing informational and adjustment counseling to families of infants and young children with hearing loss birth to 5 years of age [Guidelines]. Available from http://www.asha.org/policy. Reprinted with permission from ASHA.

Audiologic Assessment of Children From Birth to 5 Years of Age fulfill the need for more specific procedures and protocols for serving young children with hearing loss across all settings. The guidelines within this document are intended to facilitate the critical role audiologists assume when providing family-focused counseling within the context of pediatric hearing health care service delivery.

It is recommended that individuals who practice independently in this area hold the Certificate of Clinical Competence in Audiology and hold a valid state license where required by law. Additionally, ASHA certified audiologists abide by the ASHA Code of Ethics, including Principle of Ethics II Rule B, which states "Individuals shall engage in only those aspects of the profession that are within their competence, considering their level of education, training, and experience."

The Guidelines for Audiologists Providing Informational and Adjustment Counseling to Families of Infants and Young Children With Hearing Loss Birth to 5 Years of Age were developed by an ASHA working group and approved by the ASHA Board of Directors in February 2008. The members of the working group responsible for the development of these guidelines were Pam Mason (ex officio), Allan O. Diefendorf (chair), Judith S. Gravel, David M. Luterman, Noel D. Matkin, Amy McConkey Robbins, and Anne Marie Tharpe. Roberta Aungst, vice president for professional practice in audiology (2004–2006), and Gwendolyn Wilson, vice president for professional practice in audiology (2007–2009), served as the monitoring vice president.

Introduction

The American Speech-Language-Hearing Association (ASHA) documents entitled Guidelines for the Audiologic Assessment of Children From Birth to 5 Years of Age (ASHA, 2004a) and Roles, Knowledge, and Skills: Audiologists Providing Clinical Services to Infants and Young Children Birth to 5 Years of Age (ASHA, 2006) emphasize the complex and unique nature of providing audiologic services to infants and young children and their families.[1] These documents advocate a continuous process of family-focused service delivery, where audiologists are simultaneously engaged in:

- Overseeing early identification (screening) programs (Joint Committee on Infant Hearing [JCIH], 2007);
- Establishing an accurate diagnosis of hearing loss (ASHA, 2004a);
- Coordinating timely audiologic services (ASHA, 2006); and,
- Providing effective family support and counseling.

The JCIH Year 2007 Position Statement: Principles and Guidelines for Early Hearing Detection and Intervention Programs (JCIH, 2007), also policy of ASHA, advocates principles that provide guidance for effective early hearing loss detection and intervention (EHDI) programs. Furthermore, the principles underlying JCIH position statements have been advocated for more than 25 years (JCIH, 1982, 1991, 1994, 2000) and are the bases for successful EHDI outcomes. Included in these principles are the following:

- All infants should have access to hearing screening using a physiologic measure at no later than 1 month of age.
- All infants who do not pass the initial hearing screening and any subsequent rescreening should have appropriate audiologic and medical evaluations to confirm the presence of hearing loss at no later than 3 months of age.
- All infants with confirmed permanent hearing loss should receive early intervention services as soon as possible after diagnosis but no later than 6 months of age.

These benchmarks must be balanced with the reality that issues related to medically compromised/fragile infants, individual coping styles, family systems, and cultural differences may not always permit adherence to these guidelines (Matkin, 1998). In addition, families with limited resources (e.g., family support, financial stability, spiritual beliefs, effective communication) will often experience challenges in moving through an EHDI system in a timely fashion. Yet, through effective counseling, support services, and sensitivity to the implications of those challenges on the parents and child, audiologists can facilitate families' abilities to adhere to a timely management plan.

This document is the third in a series of practice policy documents (ASHA, 2004a, 2006). These guidelines are intended to provide audiologists with information about supporting and counseling families that facilitates successful outcomes for those families being served by EHDI programs. Furthermore, this document is based on the premise that families desire and require relevant information, support, and individualized recommendations throughout the screening, diagnostic, and intervention process (Harrison & Roush, 2002).

Prior to the 1990s, infants with severe and profound hearing loss were identified at around 2 to 2½ years of age (National Institutes of Health, 1993; U.S. Department of Health and Human Services, Public Health Service, 1990). For children with lesser degrees of bilateral and unilateral hearing loss, the age of identification was often as late as school entry. Furthermore, identification was typically initiated by parents concerned about their child's auditory responses, their lack of or delay in speech and language development, or their poor performance in school.

Early identification paradigms have changed considerably because of the recognized benefits of early detection of hearing loss within the first year of life (e.g., Kennedy et al., 2006; Moeller, 2000; Yoshinago-Itano, Sedey, Coulter, & Mehl, 1998). Remarkable improvements in communication and developmental outcomes can be largely attributed to advances in the technologies available for detecting and diagnosing hearing loss, as well as those used for intervention, including amplification incorporating sophisticated signal processing capabilities and cochlear implants. Consequently, parents are no longer likely to be initiating the identification process. Rather, almost 99% of birthing hospitals in the United States provide, either by state mandate or voluntarily, early detection of hearing loss through "universal" newborn hearing screening programs. In turn, audiologists are confirming the newborn hearing screening result often within the first few months of life, and thereafter providing support throughout the EHDI process.

Yet, prior to audiologic confirmation of permanent hearing loss and certainly thereafter, families in contemporary society readily access health information through a variety of sources, including the Internet. It is now frequently the case that audiologists no longer select the information to provide to families, but rather filter the vast amounts of information (both helpful and potentially detrimental) that families bring with them to clinical appointments. These changes in the timing of early screening for hearing loss, information access, and subsequent accelerated service provision require an expanded set of counseling skills by audiologists.

This context necessitates that family-focused information and emotional support counseling be infused into all interactions with families during the EHDI process and within every opportunity for pediatric audiologic practice thereafter. As such, family-focused counseling is not a separate service or event. In supplying information and support to families, audiologists recognize and respond to families' emotional needs following newborn hearing screening, at the time of the confirmation of the hearing loss, and throughout childhood.

The ultimate goal of these clinical interactions is to support the development of informed, independent, and empowered families. To achieve this outcome, audiologists judiciously provide information and guidance and, as needed, emotional support. To this end, parents' questions and comments guide the quantity of information needed, the level of detail provided, and the amount of emotional support required (Luterman, 2006b).

As seen in Figure A–1, audiologists initially provide substantial emotional support so that families can gain emotional strength. At the same time, audiologists are providing informational counseling so as to increase parental knowledge and competency as they grow to become strong advocates for their children.

The roles of audiologists transition over time to those of facilitator and advocate. Audiologists strive to balance these roles

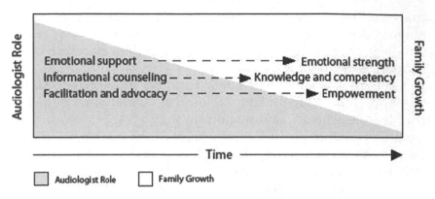

Figure A–1. Audiologist role in family growth.

while concurrently promoting family independence. Ultimately, the family becomes empowered to be the primary decision maker for their child.

Scope

The scope of this document is intended to facilitate family-focused counseling for parents and caregivers of children with hearing loss from birth to 5 years of age by audiologists as a routine and valued component of their clinical practice. Family-focused counseling provides emotional support to parents and caregivers as they adjust to the child's hearing loss, and informational counseling supports them as they learn about the myriad of audiologic, developmental, psychosocial, communication, and educational implications of permanent childhood hearing loss. It is important to note that counseling remains dynamic while it is infused into all aspects of service delivery, sometimes comprising information dissemination and exchange (content counseling), and sometimes involving the provision of emotional support. Throughout the child's formative years, counseling is an integral part of comprehensive service provision.

Terminology

Informational Counseling

Informational counseling is the imparting of information to families about a broad range of topics throughout childhood, including, but not limited to, the following:

- Audiogram interpretation
- Amplification/technology options
- Educational options
- Communication options
- Advocacy and public health and education policies

The audiologist's challenge is to provide sufficient information to assist families in decision making. Clear, concise explanations and information are needed. Terminology that misleads or confuses parents may influence a family's acceptance of hearing loss and postpone or at least delay the implementation of needed services. Additionally, audiologists are continually balancing education and guidance with their role as facilitator and advocate for informed decision making by families.

Adjustment to Hearing Loss Counseling

Given an appropriate support system, families can grow and change. Furthermore, families can and do directly influence their children's outcomes. Therefore, time and effort directed at the family during the EHDI process will likely result in family growth that can benefit the child over time (DeConde Johnson, 1997). Adjustment to hearing loss counseling refers to the support provided by audiologists to families as they learn of their child's hearing loss and attempt to recognize, acknowledge, and understand the realities of having a child with hearing loss.

It is within the scope of practice in audiology to infuse emotional support during interactions with families (ASHA, 2004b). Yet, audiologists must be vigilant in observing the few parents who demonstrate severe emotional responses to their child's diagnosis, particularly when those responses continue for lengthy periods of time and/or become more acute over time. In such cases, the parent's need for counseling or other supports may be beyond the scope of practice for audiologists, who should then be prepared to refer families to appropriate mental health care professionals.

Family Focused

Family-focused service provision attempts to achieve a balance between a systems- and technology-driven approach to EHDI. Although current public policy supported by scientific evidence endorses timely progression from identification of hearing loss to intervention (JCIH, 2007), it is recognized that not all families can or will be able to comply with recommended benchmarks. Families do not process or accept new information with equal speed and accuracy. Therefore, regardless of the age of identification, the implementation of intervention services should progress at the family's desired pace. The desires and needs of the family must be acknowledged and supported, and given equally high priority as any public or institutional policy, keeping in mind that families are their children's primary decision makers and change agents. That is, throughout the diagnostic and early decision-making process and, later, as the individualized family service plan (IFSP) is developed, the family decides a course of action that best meets their family's needs at these critical points in time.

The impact on and/or influence of a family's cultural background also should be considered during assessment and intervention services provision. Potential linguistic and cultural barriers to interacting with families must be identified and a plan developed to address these needs. This helps to ensure effective communication and follow-up. Culturally and linguistically appropriate modes of communication, which may include the use of interpreters or translators, should be used during assessment and management (Scott, 2002).

Families should be actively involved in the assessment and intervention process to the extent they desire and to the extent feasible given the complex nature of audiologic service delivery. The family's rights (including informed consent and confidentiality issues), reasonable expectations, reasonable needs, and preferences are paramount and must be considered throughout the provision of services. Additionally, EHDI systems must honor racial, ethnic, cultural, and socioeconomic diversity of families.

Unbiased Information

This document advocates the concept that families make informed choices for all aspects of their children's communication and educational development. Optimally, decision making is based on the best information that is available at the time, which the family receives through the audiologist as well as other sources. These decisions are made as families weigh the information they receive along with their desires for their child. Unbiased implies that only families are in the position to decide what outcomes they want for their children. Unbiased also implies that information provided to families is delivered in a straightforward manner without filters or hidden agendas. Providing unbiased information requires a recognition and revelation of one's own biases and opinions, fully disclosing any biases to families by stating the same, and then providing a basis for the opinion.

It is important to remember that the term unbiased does not imply that audiologists cannot or should not offer their expert opinions to families. Indeed, decisions families make are facilitated by the information provided by audiologists regarding, for example, the specifics of the child's hearing loss and amplification and communication options. This input is valued by and critical to families as they consider the myriad of choices and decisions that EHDI systems afford (Harrison & Roush, 2002). Once families are ready to make informed decisions about desired outcomes, audiologists are then obligated to inform families on how best to achieve those outcomes.

Best practice is based on several premises that require audiologists to have firsthand, current knowledge of (a) published studies, including outcomes research and guidelines that support evidence-based practice; (b) children having a wide range of hearing loss (this implies that audiologists need to have a broad range of clinical experience); (c) auditory development and opportunities afforded by amplification and implantable devices technologies; (d) early intervention and educational practices and opportunities; and (e) public health and education law. All of these pieces of information are of great worth to families. It is the clinician's responsibility when counseling families to separate biased views from professional delivery of up-to-date information, and to ensure that families know the difference.

Family Stress

Depression is a common stress-related response for hearing parents of children with hearing loss. Evidence suggests that mothers are more inclined than fathers to experience depression in response to their child's hearing loss (Mavrolas, 1990; Meadow-Orlans, 1995; Prior, Glazner, Sanson, & Debelle, 1988). Maternal depression places children with hearing loss at additional risk for emotional, communication, and cognitive difficulties, because of the implications for emotional availability and effective interactions between mothers and children (Cohn, Campbell, Matias, & Hopkins, 1990; Field et al., 1988; Radke-Yarrow, 1998). Watson, Henggeler, and Whelan (1990) were able to show that a lack of social competence in hard of hearing youths occurred in correlation with parental stress experience. Increased behavioral problems were associated with poor emotional adaptation and a generally stressed family situation.

In a classic contribution to the field, Green and Solnit (1964) recognized more than 40 years ago that some parents with children having chronic conditions have a tendency to overprotect and overindulge their children, leading to overly dependent children and compromised developmental progress. For example, parents may harbor long-term fears that their "vulnerable child" (Green & Solnit, 1964) will experience "changes" in hearing over time.

Grieving also may be a common response of parents who have just learned about their child's hearing loss. Parental grieving may occur at various times in the EHDI process, during the early school-age years, and throughout the active years of parenting. That is, grief is a complex and evolving emotional response that is internalized differently and triggered differently at various times throughout the time span of parenting a child with hearing loss. Additionally, grieving will not occur in an orderly manner or have a finite endpoint. As such, it is more realistic to consider various emotions as reflecting different states rather than different stages of grief. Often in a Western culture our manner of rational thinking is linear, yet the grief and healing process may be better considered as it is in Native American cultures. That is, grieving and healing can best be illustrated not as a straight ascending line but as a circular, yet upward, spiral (Figure A–2).

Although families learn to cope with adversity over time, they still revisit old concerns and experience old feelings, but often with better developed coping skills and with greater cognitive awareness. In other words, grief is chronic and continues to be triggered by unexpected events and at different times.

Applying Information and Adjustment Counseling to the EHDI Process

The following sections reflect stages in the EHDI process that are considered to be critical in the transition of families as they

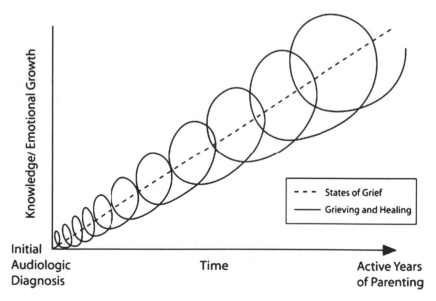

Figure A–2. Grieving and healing.

integrate children into their family structure and culture. In turn, the following sections of this guidelines document propose recommendations for best practices for counseling families made on the basis of best data available, while recognizing that evidence for any specific counseling approach is currently limited.

Newborn Hearing Screening

Informational Counseling

Audiologists are involved with all aspects of early identification of hearing loss, including program development, staff training, coordination, management, assessment of program quality, oversight of outpatient referral, and reducing lost to follow-up (JCIH, 2007). Audiologists are the most qualified professionals to provide ongoing training and oversight of hospital nursery staff relative to the newborn hearing screening process (JCIH, 2007). As such, and to the extent possible, audiologists should be the professionals who communicate with parents when a baby has not passed a hearing screening. However, it is recognized that within certain medical settings audiologists may not be available to convey the results before hospital discharge. Under those circumstances, audiologists ensure that others (such as nurses, technicians, or physicians) provide screening outcomes in oral and written forms and in a sensitive and considerate manner.

To facilitate this process, in-service education should always include information about how hearing screening results are presented to families, assuring that parents understand the reasons that a failure might occur in the nursery, appreciate the need to promptly follow-up with further screening or audiologic testing, and that early hearing loss detection often occurs over multiple clinical visits.

The following principles support effective informational counseling:

- Communication with parents is confidential and presented in a family-focused manner.
- Information is delivered in a clear and concise manner avoiding technical jargon.

- Parents are given the opportunity and encouragement to ask questions.

Initial information in verbal and written forms and in the language used by families in the home should include:

- The rationale for screening of the newborn for hearing loss;
- A description of screening procedure(s) and possible outcomes;
- Explanations for a failed screening outcome and its implications;
- The importance of prompt follow up (ASHA, 1996, 2004a; JCIH, 2007); and,
- Reasons why additional testing might be needed.

It is important to remember that if information about the screening process is provided only after a mother is admitted to the hospital to deliver her child, she may not have the level of concentration needed to consider adequately the information being presented. Therefore, it is recommended that educational materials also be:

- Provided as part of hospital prenatal education programs and/or public health clinic outreach programs;
- Written at a 4th to 5th grade literacy level; and,
- Available in the preferred language of the family.

As already noted, recommendations for follow-up audiologic services (i.e., second stage outpatient rescreen and/or direct referral for testing by an audiologist) should be delivered in person to the parents by the audiologist. Use of the phrase "referral for further testing" rather than the term "failure" is more sensitive language and less alarming for conveying screening results and recommendations. Presenting these findings in a positive manner that emphasizes their importance may help to ensure that recommendations for additional testing are followed. Because of mitigating circumstances, communicating this information to parents of children in the well-baby nursery may be different than communicating the same results to parents of children who have extended stays in the NICU. If follow-up is needed, families should receive:

- Explicit recommendations on how to secure follow-up testing, including names and phone numbers of follow-up screening facilities;
- An audiologist to whom to direct questions in the interim; and,
- Local, state, and national resources to obtain information regarding subsequent stages of the EHDI process

Additionally, although the goal of universal newborn hearing screening is to identify all infants with developmentally significant hearing loss, it is recognized that some children with minimal to mild degrees of hearing loss and unusual configurations of hearing loss will pass the newborn hearing screening (Johnson et al., 2005). Similarly, children who experience late-onset hearing loss (Fortnum, 2003) also are likely to pass newborn screening (JCIH, 2007). When children have passed a newborn screening and at a later date are diagnosed with permanent types of hearing loss, this may complicate acceptance of the diagnosis by some families. Therefore, despite passing a newborn hearing screening or when families choose to not participate in screening, parents should be counseled about the need for ongoing surveillance and periodic monitoring of auditory and speech-language skills throughout early childhood (JCIH, 2000, 2007).

Adjustment Counseling

Despite advances in screening technology and undeniable advantages of early intervention for hearing loss, there are emotional challenges associated with the newborn screening process for families (Tharpe & Clayton, 1997). Consider that because of the advent of universal newborn hearing screening, parents are receiving unsolicited information about the program and their infant's hearing screening outcome at a sensitive and potentially vulnerable time. Consistent with informed consent and ethical practice, parents should be informed through verbal and written information that their newborn's hearing will be screened prior to hospital discharge, and screening outcomes also must be communicated. Parents should have the opportunity to opt out of the hearing screening for personal or religious reasons. Regardless, it is important to provide support counseling at this sensitive and emotionally fragile stage of the EHDI process. Adjustment counseling for families whose infants have failed a screening may include listening and responding to fears or concerns expressed by families, and ensuring follow-up of the failed screening in a timely manner to ameliorate stress and anxiety in families.

The timing of receipt of screening results coupled with the manner in which this information is conveyed has the potential to interfere with parent-child bonding, which is essential to the mental health of children (Gregory, 1999, 2001). Therefore, this is a critical juncture in the identification process and might well determine whether parents comply with the recommendation for further assessment.

There might be occasional circumstances when hearing screening at a later time would be more appropriate for some families (Eichwald, 2007; Luterman, 2007; Young & Tattersall, 2007). A small percentage of parents may refuse the in-hospital hearing screening, and, particularly in cases of the medically fragile NICU infants, families may choose to defer hearing screening. Under these circumstances, information about hearing screening, hearing loss, developmental milestones, and the availability of hearing screening after hospital discharge should be provided. Families should be supported in whatever decision they make regarding the screening process. However, families also should be made aware that in some states data on babies missed and/or those who refuse the hospital-based newborn hearing screening are reported to the state (National Center for Hearing Assessment and Management, 2007).

Despite these challenges, there is evidence that the majority of parents of children with normal hearing and hearing loss desire newborn hearing screening and recognize the importance of early detection of hearing loss even when parents experience stress and anxiety at the time of diagnosis (Barringer, Mauk, Jensen, & Woods-Kershner, 1997; Davis et al., 2006; Luterman & Kurtzer-White, 1999; Watkin, Beckman, & Baldwin, 1995). Therefore, the importance of coupling the screening process with parent information and support is crucial for facilitating smooth and timely transitions to the diagnostic process. Personnel involved in screening programs should be vigilant about improving outcomes (decreasing both the false positive and false negative rates), enhancing the manner and content of information provided to families, and optimizing the timing, delivery, and quality of information from the newborn hearing screening (Arnold et al., 2006; Davis et al., 2006).

Confirmation of Hearing Loss

Informational Counseling

An audiologist is typically the first and most desired professional who bears the responsibility for describing the hearing loss and its implications to family members (Harrison & Roush, 2002; Luterman & Kurtzer-White, 1999). This responsibility requires audiologists to be knowledgeable, skilled, and experienced in providing information that might be upsetting, stress-evoking, and even painful for some families. Equally important is the follow-up emotional support, guidance, and education that must be provided to families (Matkin, 1988). It is important to remember that it is at this point in service delivery where individualized continuity of care by an audiologist is initiated.

In the initial stages of diagnosis and confirmation of hearing loss, the audiologist will need to assume a substantial role in providing information and explaining procedures for assessing hearing in children. This may include the following:

- Reasons why sleeping during testing is desirable for some tests, but not others;
- Reasons for the use of moderate sedation to achieve optimal test conditions and why medical monitoring of the child's health status is required;
- Explanations of different test procedures and why each is important; and,
- Explanations for why some tests may need to be repeated periodically.

Sharing audiometric results is a routine matter to audiologists, and frequently the initial interactions with families take on the effect of a rehearsed verbal template, in which the details of complex tests are explained in lay terminology. Although a necessary component of the counseling process, this imparting of test results, or informational counseling, can be perceived by the listener as a way of maintaining an uncaring professional distance. Beazely and Moore (1995) have discussed this in terms of "wearing an expert mantle" rather than making genuine, heartfelt contact. It is recommended that initially, audiometric results be explained to families in functional terms. In other words, families need to understand the impact of the hearing loss on a child's development more than the axes on the audiogram and hearing levels in decibels.

Because 90% or more of infants with hearing loss are born to hearing parents, most families have very little knowledge of childhood hearing loss. Furthermore, some parents may still be integrating their baby into the family unit with natural uncertainty and insecurity. Yet, families do possess parental instincts and a developing knowledge of their child and should be enlisted as collaborators in all aspects of the diagnostic process rather than being treated as passive participants. It is well established that involvement of families in the provision of clinical services is crucial for families' acceptance of hearing loss (Luterman, 1999). Collaboration may include active roles such as:

- Shaping the priorities and objectives of the visit;
- Providing descriptions of their childs auditory behaviors, either through conversation or completion of questionnaires;
- Sharing observations of their child's development and behavior;
- Participating with the child in demonstration of skills or compliance with the test battery; and,
- Providing feedback on the child's behavior throughout the behavioral audiologic test battery (i.e., how representative was the behavior of the child?).

A family's presence and/or participation allows the audiologist to explain the purpose of each step of the assessment, which in turn improves the family's ability to understand the findings of an otherwise abstract and technical test process.

It is recommended that during the confirmation of hearing loss:

- Follow-up testing to confirm the initial diagnostic impression be scheduled as soon as possible to minimize the family's concern during the diagnostic phase; when possible, audiologists contact families ahead of time to explain the upcoming tests;
- All diagnostic testing be conducted by the same audiologist in order to enhance continuity of care, encourage the development of rapport and trust, and minimize the likelihood of receiving different interpretations of the results from different audiologists;
- Parents' questions and comments guide the quantity of information and the level of detail provided; and,
- Audiologists provide time for parents to discuss their problems and concerns.

Adjustment to Hearing Loss Counseling

Audiologists should be aware that first impressions may set the tone for subsequent interactions with families. Therefore, a positive and respectful attitude is a necessary first step for developing an effective rapport with families. Respect includes sensitivity to nontraditional family structures, socioeconomic circumstances, cultural diversity, and differing viewpoints, regardless of whether those views are mutually embraced or whether realities are completely understood. Once rapport and respect are established, a sense of trust can evolve, which is strengthened as the relationship continues. The audiologist allows for the time necessary to establish such trusting relationships, even at the risk of creating slight delays in the diagnostic process.

Adjustment to hearing loss counseling by audiologists at this important juncture may include the following:

- Recognizing a family's fragility during the EHDI process;
- Recognizing the impact of the diagnosis of hearing loss on a family, including the child's siblings, grandparents, and other extended family members;

- Identifying family supports (e.g., friends, clergy) and encouraging families to seek their assistance when needed;
- Focusing on the family's strengths and special needs within the context of their cultural and value systems;
- Recognizing the difference between acute grief and clinical depression, and making appropriate referrals; and,
- Providing emotional support.

For counseling to be most effective, informational and adjustment counseling must be balanced. Although families will need information to facilitate decision making, many times families are not requesting information, but rather are expressing an emotional or affective concern about their child's recently identified hearing loss. That is, many times a family's message or questions will contain both content and affective components, and deciding which component requires priority is critical in developing a trusting relationship. The ability to distinguish content from affective components is referred to as "differentiation" (Cormier & Hackney, 1999). It is one of the primary learning objectives in counselor education and is essential in the developing relationship between audiologists and families. Cormier and Hackney advocated that audiologists' responses should reflect the patient's or families' intent. That is, when a family requests information, the audiologist should respond with information, and when a family expresses an emotion, the audiologist should let the family know that the emotion was acknowledged and respected.

By having their emotional needs addressed, families may be more amenable to new information and more likely to make informed decisions. Yet, some audiologists may feel compelled to protect families from emotional reactions after receiving unexpected, upsetting, and potentially stress-evoking information (Luterman, 2001). Any effort to rescue families (i.e., to imply the audiologist's approach guarantees a positive outcome) should be avoided, as this may actually foster dependency. Families need to progress at their own rates through various stages of personal adjustment.

An awareness of the stages of grief as a response to hearing loss is not sufficient for understanding a family's reaction to the confirmation of hearing loss. That is, Luterman (2006a) noted that the grief reaction of parents to the identification of hearing loss is not similar to the loss of a loved one to death. In death, there is finality to the grief; there is a burial and life can go on, albeit with pain and loss. With hearing loss, grief can be chronic, lived every hour of every day. The child may be a constant reminder to the parents of this loss. No matter how well adjusted the parents seem to be to the reality that their child has a hearing loss, there can be trigger events (e.g., child's birthday party, anniversary of their original diagnostic evaluation, individualized education program [IEP] meetings) that remind them of the loss and those initial feelings of pain and sorrow may return.

In some cases, grief associated with the diagnosis of hearing loss in children may result in clinical depression in parents. It is important for audiologists to recognize the signs of clinical depression, as opposed to acute grief, to help identify which families would benefit from referral to a mental health professional. The clinical signs of depression include:

- Not keeping appointments;
- Deep feelings of sadness;
- Difficulty thinking, concentrating, remembering, or making decisions;
- Feelings of hopelessness, pessimism;
- Loss of energy or increased fatigue;
- Insomnia; and,
- Withdrawal/isolation from family.

Providing emotional support to families involves different communication skills than informational counseling, including the ability to talk less, listen more, and listen actively (English, Lucks, Rojeski, & Hornak, 1999). Clinicians need not be afraid of periods of silence, tears, or expressions of anger. Silence may be a time when parents are attempting to integrate and think about their feelings and it is important that parent silence not be interrupted. Audiologists need to be comfortable with the silence and allow families this time. Tears also are a natural expression of grief. The simple act of handing a tissue to a distressed parent is a silent form of acknowledgment and support of the parent's feelings.

In addition, anger is often a reflection of a family's fear, a sense of violation of expectation, and a loss of control. However, anger is not necessarily a judgment on the audiologist's competency. Provision of emotional support, despite this anger, is crucial. Audiologists must be especially sensitive to families whose vulnerability and fragility (e.g., due to extended time in NICU, chronic illness, limited parental education, concurrent family stressors) necessitates extra time for them to understand and accept their child's hearing loss. Recognizing a family's fragility assists in determining the rate that they can integrate and process information. This recognition can help audiologists respond sensitively and without defensiveness should they become the target of a family's anger or frustration.

Although the confirmation of hearing loss may evoke an emotional response, the audiologist should view this response as a revealing affective component in the evolving counseling process. The establishment of a positive professional relationship can bring comfort to families during this stressful time. Audiologists also should recognize that the magnitude of the hearing loss is not a predictor of the extent of the parental stress response. Regardless of the degree of hearing loss, it is the parent's perception of the problem that dictates the amount of support needed.

Lederberg and Golbach (2002) found a difference in the stress experience of parents with deaf and hard of hearing children at age 2 years but not at age 3. Early diagnosis and intervention appear to be the best prevention strategy against stress for the parents of deaf and hard of hearing children.

Intervention and Habilitation

Informational Counseling

Audiologists are responsible for providing families with unbiased information, recommendations, and appropriate educational and communication options based on family decisions and informed choices. As such, audiologists are responsible to families and not for families.

Children with hearing loss, even those with similar audiograms, represent a heterogeneous population. These children and their families will come to audiologists with a wide range of concerns. Listening to families about their hopes and desires for their children will guide this process. Informational counseling to families might include:

- Communication options appropriate for the family's desire for spoken or visual language;
- Technology options, including candidacy for cochlear implants;
- The range of educational options appropriate to their child's hearing loss and developmental needs, including encouraging families to observe intervention programs on-site;
- Provision of information relative to the importance of ongoing monitoring and verification of amplification;
- Hearing aid orientation, troubleshooting, and maintenance for families, other caregivers, speech-language pathologists, educators/early interventionists, and the child when appropriate;
- Long-term audiologic follow-up, including addressing questions of progressive hearing loss;
- Processes associated with educational transitions;
- Public law and advocacy relevant to public education and public access; and,
- Other informational resources including, but not limited to, Web sites, printed materials, and DVDs.

During this time, communication among the audiologist, the child's medical home (American Academy of Pediatrics, 2005), and child's family is essential for securing appropriate services (JCIH, 2007). This also might help avoid confusion from conflicting information or recommendations received from various allied professionals.

Audiologists should encourage parents to acknowledge and celebrate the capabilities, as well as the special needs, of their children. By the late preschool years, children should be included as much as possible in feedback and decision making in their own management. This will initially consist of small steps (e.g., selecting the color of their hearing aids, learning to check their hearing aid batteries) that can lead to enhanced self-esteem and greater independence.

An additional responsibility of audiologists is to advocate for the development of quality educational options within their communities. Currently, family decisions are too often based solely on availability of services; that is, selecting from a limited number of services rather than the selection of their most desired option for communication and education. Therefore, audiologists should advocate for the establishment of diagnostic teaching facilities and a range of educational options, if not available, within the community. In addition, it is important that audiologists participate on multidisciplinary management teams with emphasis on facilitating communication, social-emotional, and cognitive development and, later, academic performance. It also is important for audiologists to participate in the IFSP and, later, the IEP processes. As families increasingly become empowered to serve as effective advocates for their children (refer to Figure A–1), the role of the audiologist as care coordinator should begin to shift to facilitator (ASHA, 2006).

Adjustment to Hearing Loss Counseling

The infusion of counseling into all interactions with families, mentioned earlier in this document, is especially important at this juncture. With an expanding array of technologies, educational options, and communication modes, families are faced with making complex decisions very early in the intervention process. They will need information relative to a range of options provided in an unbiased, supportive manner.

Intervention should be provided with sensitivity to the family's readiness to proceed. There may be a wide time range of when families are ready to proceed with intervention. That is, some families come into the process with strong coping skills and extensive support structures allowing them to move forward in a timely manner.

Scorgie, Wilgosh, and McDonald (1998) summarized the most important variables for understanding the coping process under four headings:

- Family variables (e.g., family socioeconomic status, cohesion, hardiness, problem-solving skills/creativity, roles and responsibilities, and composition);
- Parent variables (e.g., quality of marital relationship, maternal locus of control, appraisal, and time/schedule concerns);
- Child variables (e.g., degree of disability, age, gender, and temperament); and,
- External variables (e.g., stigmatizing social attitudes, social network supports, and collaboration with professionals).

Calderon and Greenberg (1993), as well as Calderon, Greenberg, and Kusche (1991), were able to show that successful coping on the mother's part has a significant influence on child development. The more successful the mothers were in acquiring helpful strategies for coping with their deaf child, the better developed the children's emotional sensitivity, reading competence, and problem-solving behavior. The children also exhibited less impulsive behavior, higher cognitive flexibility, and better social competence.

Webster-Stratton (1990) pointed out another crucial aspect of coping that demonstrates the close correlation between parental experience and parental behavior: Specifically, there was a close association between reported parental stress and more frequent use of punishment, discipline, and constraint in day-to-day parenting.

When families lack resources to engage in even the most basic aspects of service delivery, audiologists must consider the number and types of demands they make on families. Awareness of the challenges each family unit faces should guide the audiologist's expectations on the family's capacity to fully follow through with an early intervention plan. Thus, a lack of follow through with the audiologist's recommendations during this time may reflect a variety of underlying causes and should not be misconstrued as a lack of caring or, as is sometimes suggested, constituting child neglect.

Audiologists must balance their information counseling with families regarding the use of hearing technologies (e.g., digital hearing aids, cochlear implants, or FM systems), with the family's perceived enticement to technology as a "cure." Although current technology has greatly ameliorated the impact of hearing loss, technology provision alone is not sufficient to the habilitation/ intervention process. The temptation to consider technology (particularly cochlear implants) as a cure for deafness should be resisted, as this diminishes the challenges still ahead and ignores the need of families to spend time resolving their loss. At the same time, audiologists recognize when families are in need of information and support in exploring their options and opportunities for their children. Facilitating families' knowledge of options and opportunities sends a hopeful message of optimism and may prevent feelings of fear and isolation.

As intervention plans are initiated, it is important that both audiologists and families recognize that all decisions are subject to change over time. Although continuity of intervention is recognized as an important factor for successful outcomes, families should always be made aware that their initial choices are amendable.

Children might require a period of diagnostic teaching to inform this process. In a diagnostic teaching approach, appropriate individual goals are set, but the interventionist continually monitors the factors that are favorable or unfavorable to a child's learning. The focus of such an approach is prominently on the positive aspect of the question: "What are the techniques and supports that help this child learn most efficiently?" Diagnostic teaching allows for the determination of effectiveness of hearing technology options that may include hearing aids, cochlear implantation, and assistive devices. Moreover, the diagnostic teaching period allows for the determination of an effective method of communication and one preferred and used continually by all members of the family. Some families and children will best be served by auditory/oral approaches (speaking and listening) to communicate while others may require a system with visual supports. Diagnostic teaching also may reveal the presence of additional disabilities not previously identified (Gallaudet Research Institute, Office of Demographic Studies, 2001).

A rich source of support for families may be found in their relationships with other families of children with hearing loss. Efforts should be made to provide families with formal and informal opportunities to meet and interact with other families with similar experiences when they desire such opportunities. Optimally, these are informed choices families make about when and which interactions would be most beneficial to them. Therefore, adjustment to hearing loss counseling in intervention and habilitation may include:

- Provision of opportunities both formal and informal to meet and interact with other families of children with hearing loss. The type of interactions that individual families choose will be based on their need for information and their desires to learn more about one or more different communication and education options. These could include introductions to culturally Deaf, oral deaf, and hard of hearing adults who use different communication modes and technology;
- Opportunities to observe children and interact with young children who use various communication approaches and technologies; and,
- Development and facilitation of family support groups.

The audiologist's role in family support groups is one of facilitator, rather than instructor. Within family support groups, parents can validate each other's experiences in ways that audiologists cannot. This interaction also can lead to growing parental empowerment as information is shared among families. All family members, including grandparents and siblings, can benefit from attending such sessions or participating in support groups that focus on shared experiences of individuals with similar roles, rather than passively listening to information provided by professionals.

In supplying information to families, audiologists should recognize and respect the family's complex (and often recurring) feelings through the grieving process, not only at the time of initial diagnosis of hearing loss, but also at different intervention decision-making stages and transitions, and throughout the active years of parenting. That is, stress is a complex and evolving emotional response that is internalized differently and triggered differently at various times throughout the time span of parenting a child with hearing loss (Luterman, 2006a).

Audiologists should be aware that families may be fearful that every subsequent audiologic assessment beyond the initial diagnosis has the potential of revealing additional difficulties or changes (decrements) in hearing threshold levels. Even families that have previously demonstrated excellent coping skills may need additional support upon learning that their child's hearing loss has progressed (Brookhouser, Worthington, & Kelly, 1994). Furthermore, there is an important role for the audiologist in supporting families with the transition of their children from early intervention to preschool and through to the school-age years.

Professional Preparation Concerns and Recommendations

Counseling in audiology has historically employed a medical model with an emphasis on providing content/informational counseling, and rarely providing emotional support. Additionally, over the past decade a medical model has served as the foundation for implementing a systems-driven paradigm (mandated universal newborn hearing screening) stressing diagnosis and intervention of hearing loss in the first 6 months of life, and providing parents and caregivers with information on the screening, follow-up, and intervention components of early detection.

Another change that has had an impact on service delivery is our nation's growing population diversity, requiring knowledge of and experience with multicultural counseling to respond to linguistic and cultural differences prevalent in the United States. As such, achieving benchmarks (i.e., positive language outcomes) in early detection is facilitated when family counseling and emotional support are actively infused into audiologic care within a systems-driven paradigm.

Professionals increasingly have become aware that family-focused counseling and instruction needs to be an integral component of screening, diagnosis, and intervention, employing the ongoing infusion concept already described. Because of the wide range of emotions associated with hearing loss, the need for formal and practical education in counseling seems apparent. Historically, preparation for addressing the emotional and personal needs of families has been limited (Martin, Barr, & Bernstein, 1992; Martin, Krall, & O'Neal, 1989). However, the current Knowledge and Skills Acquisition Summary Form (ASHA, 2003) provides a general acknowledgement of this need. More specific recommendations for the preparation of audiologists to provide counseling include the following:

- Explicit coursework in curricula—expand traditional view of counseling to include dealing with emotional impact of diagnosis of childhood hearing loss on families:
  - Knowledge of child development and necessary parenting skills as essential prerequisites to management;
  - Knowledge of the grieving process and the role that emotional states play in the acceptance process;
  - Knowledge of personal adjustment counseling;
  - Knowledge of family systems theory;
  - Knowledge of cultural differences; and,
  - Knowledge of the impact of limited resources (e.g., financial, emotional) on a family's ability to cope with a stressor such as hearing loss.
- Practical observation and supervised experience with:
  - Families with children of different ages in clinical and informal settings;
  - Families in different stages of acceptance;
  - Families at different points in the service delivery continuum;
  - Family support groups; and,
  - Mentor counselors.

Appropriate counseling is a critical variable in the habilitation/rehabilitation of individuals with hearing loss (see Crandell, 1997, and Luterman, 2001, for a review of these investigations). Yet, historically, little has been done to equip audiologists with these skills. McCarthy, Culpepper, and Lucks (1986) found that only 12% of university communication disorders programs in the United States offered coursework and practice in counseling. Almost 10 years later, the authors repeated their study and found essentially no change (Culpepper, Mendel, & McCarthy, 1994).

Similarly, Crandell (1997) examined the availability of counseling instruction with audiology graduate programs. Results indicated that less than one half of the programs offered a counseling course. Moreover, only 27% of the audiology departments that offered a counseling course required that course to be taken. Because of this lack of required course work, programs estimated that only 18% of their students ever took a counseling course prior to graduation. With the recent transition of the entry level degree from a master's to a clinical doctorate plus additional required course work, this dearth in counseling education may be, at least, partially remediated. However, it will be important for professional organizations such as ASHA to monitor the provision of this course work as well as postprofessional preparation in this most critical requisite to quality audiology practices with the pediatric population.

Future Research Needs

Much remains to be learned about effective counseling approaches for use with families of children with hearing loss. Every effort should be made to enhance our knowledge base in this important area. Recommended research areas include the following:

- Psychosocial effects of newborn hearing screening on the child and the family.
- Impact of false positive and false negative screening outcomes on families, including:
  - Stress factors
  - Coping mechanisms
  - Quality of life issues
- Parental understanding of content and retention of information relative to:
  - All components of the in-hospital and outpatient screening process

- A medical-based approach versus a family-centered approach and their integration
- Use of hearing aids, cochlear implants, and other assistive devices
- Speech and language development
- Parental compliance with follow-up relative to screening, assessment, and intervention:
  - Method of communicating follow-up recommendations (written vs. oral)
  - Impact of family's educational background and socioeconomic status
  - Impact of family's cultural and linguistic differences
  - Impact of NICU versus well-baby hospital stay on family's compliance with follow-up
- Key factors related to family satisfaction with services and transitioning from one to another, in particular:
  - Early intervention services
  - Preschool programs
  - Regular school system
- Factors that contribute to family fragility, such as:
  - Behavioral markers
  - Family support systems
- Predictors for successful family outcomes.
- Innovative approaches to the delivery of family counseling and support services for those who lack the resources that facilitate their ability to participate fully in the EHDI system.

Our current body of counseling literature is largely based on late identification of hearing loss in children, not our current reality of early detection in the newborn period. As such, there is a great need for more current investigations into the counseling process and its effectiveness for families with newly identified infants with hearing loss. Such studies are recommended to test the validity of current counseling practices in early identification, diagnosis, and intervention. Additionally, much information may be gleaned from parent reports, questionnaires, and structured interview schedules that, when constructed in compliance with robust research principles, yield valuable first-person data that informs what clinicians may come to view as best practice.

Summary

These guidelines were developed with the goal of infusing family-focused counseling within today's opportunities for early identification through a systems- and technology-driven model of service delivery (i.e., the 1–3–6 guidelines [Centers for Disease Control and Prevention, 2006]). Within this framework, a family's individuality and resources, diversity, cultural background, coping style, and learning style are recognized, supported, and respected. These guidelines reinforce the goals of the Joint Committee on Infant Hearing and adherence to pediatric audiologic service delivery consistent with the 1–3–6 guidelines of EHDI (Centers for Disease Control and Prevention, 2006; JCIH, 2007).

For counseling to be most effective, information counseling and adjustment counseling/emotional support must be balanced. The goal is to facilitate the development of informed, independent, and empowered families who will make good decisions for themselves and their child.

In some areas, there is a shortage of audiologists to comprehensively evaluate and appropriately manage infants and toddlers with hearing loss and counsel their families. As such, university education programs are encouraged to expand preservice curricula that address the unique knowledge and skills (ASHA, 2006) needed for working with infants and young children with hearing loss in culturally sensitive and family-centered ways. In addition, in-service education and continuing education focusing on the infusion of counseling into all aspects of service delivery for infants and young children and their families also must be encouraged.

The foundation of outcomes studies upon which EHDI policies were implemented must be expanded. To the extent possible, counseling families during crucial periods of parenting should be evidence based and outcome directed.

Notes

1. The term family includes biologic and/or adoptive parents, foster parents, grandparents, or others who live with the

child in a familial environment. Legal definitions of family may vary by jurisdiction. The title parents means the caregivers who share primary responsibilities for the child's care and welfare. Audiologists must honor all family relationships and maintain compliance with HIPAA regulations and other privacy requirements.

References

American Academy of Pediatrics. (2005). *Newborn and infant hearing screening activities.* Available from http://www.medicalhomeinfo .org

American Speech-Language-Hearing Association. (1996). *Guidelines for audiologic screening* [Guidelines]. Available from http://www.asha .org/policy

American Speech-Language-Hearing Association. (2003). *Knowledge and Skills Acquisition (KASA) Summary Form for certification in audiology.* Available from http://www.asha.org/about/membership-certification/handbooks/kasa-tips.htm

American Speech-Language-Hearing Association. (2004a). *Guidelines for the audiologic assessment of children from birth to 5 years of age* [Guidelines]. Available from http://www.asha.org/policy

American Speech-Language-Hearing Association. (2004b). *Scope of practice in audiology.* Available from http://www.asha.org/policy

American Speech-Language-Hearing Association. (2006). *Roles, knowledge, and skills: Audiologists providing clinical services to infants and young children birth to 5 years of age* [Knowledge and Skills]. Available from http://www.asha.org/policy

Arnold, C. L., Davis, T. C., Frempong, J. O., Humiston, S. G., Bocchini, A., Kennen, E. M., & Lloyd-Puryear, M. (2006). Assessment of newborn screening parent education materials. *Pediatrics, 117*(5, Pt. 2), S320–S325.

Barringer, D. G., Mauk, G. W., Jensen, S., & Woods-Kershner, N. (1997). Survey of parents' perceptions regarding hospital-based newborn screening. *Audiology Today, 9*(1), 18–19.

Beazely, S., & Moore, M. (1995). *Deaf children, their families, and professionals: Dismantling barriers.* London, UK: David Fulton.

Brookhouser, P., Worthington, D., & Kelly, W. (1994). Fluctuating and or progressive sensorineural hearing loss in children. *Laryngoscope, 104*, 958–964.

Calderon, R., & Greenberg, M. T. (1993). Considerations in adaptation of families with school-aged deaf children. In M. Marschark & M. D. Clark (Eds.), *Psychological perspectives on deafness* (pp. 27–47). Hillsdale, NJ: Erlbaum.

Calderon, R., Greenberg, M. T., & Kusche, C. (1991). The influence of family coping on the cognitive and social skills of deaf children. In D. Martin (Ed.), *Advances in cognition, education and deafness* (pp. 195–200). Washington, DC: Gallaudet University Press.

Centers for Disease Control and Prevention. (2006, October 27). *National EHDI goals.* Available from www.cdc.gov/ncbddd/ehdi/nationalgoals.htm

Cohn, J., Campbell, S., Matias, R., & Hopkins, J. (1990). Face-to-face interactions of postpartum depressed and nondepressed mother-infant pairs at two months. *Developmental Psychology, 26,* 15–23.

Cormier, S., & Hackney, H. (1999). *Counseling strategies and interventions* (5th ed.). Boston, MA: Allyn & Bacon.

Crandell, C. C. (1997). An update on counseling instruction with audiology programs. *Journal of the Academy of Rehabilitative Audiology, 15,* 77–86.

Culpepper, N. B., Mendel, L. L., & McCarthy, P. A. (1994). Counseling experiences and training offered by ESB-accredited programs: An update. *Asha, 36*(6), 55–58.

Davis, T. C., Humiston, S. G., Arnold, C. L., Bocchini, J. A., Bass, P. F., Kennen, E. M., et al. (2006). Recommendations for effective newborn screening communication: Results of focus groups with parents, providers and experts. *Pediatrics, 117*(5, Pt. 2), S326–S340.

DeConde Johnson, C. (1997). Understanding and advising parents and families. *Hearing Review,* 18–20.

Eichwald, J. (2007, July 17). Newborn hearing screening: A response to David Luterman. *The ASHA Leader, 12*(9), 24–25.

English, K., Lucks, L., Rojeski, T., & Hornak, J. (1999). Counseling in audiology, or learning to listen: Pre- and post-measures from an audiology counseling course. *American Journal of Audiology, 8,* 1–6.

Field, T., Healy, G., Goldstein, S., Perry, S., Bendell, D., Schanberg, S., et al. (1988). Infants of depressed mothers show depressed behavior even with nondepressed adults. *Child Development, 59,* 1569–1579.

Fortnum, H. M. (2003). Epidemiology of permanent childhood hearing impairment: Implications for neonatal hearing screening. *Audiologic Medicine, 1*(3), 155–164.

Gallaudet Research Institute, Office of Demographic Studies. (2001, January). *Regional and national summary report of data from 1999–2000 Annual Survey of Deaf and Hard of Hearing Children*

& Youth. Washington, DC: Author. Available from http://gri.gallaudet .edu/Demographics/

Green, M., & Solnit, A. J. (1964). Reactions to the threatened loss of a child: A vulnerable child syndrome. *Pediatrics, 34*, 58–66.

Gregory, S. (1999). *Cochlear implantation and the under 2's: Psychological and social implications.* Paper presented at the Nottingham Paediatric Implant Programme International Conference, Cochlear Implantation in the Under 2's; Research Into Clinical Practice, Nottingham, England.

Gregory, S. (2001, September). *Consensus on auditory implants.* Paper presented at the Ethical Aspects and Counseling Conference, Padova, Italy.

Harrison, M., & Roush, J. (2002). Information for families with young deaf and hard of hearing children: Reports from parents and pediatric audiologists. In R. C. Seewald & J. S. Gravel (Eds.), *A sound foundation through early amplification* (pp. 233–249). Warrenville, IL: Phonak AG.

Johnson, J. L., White, K. R., Widen, J. E., Gravel, J. S., James, M., Kennalley, T., et al. (2005). A multicenter evaluation of how many infants with permanent hearing loss pass a two-stage otoacoustic emissions/ automated auditory brainstem response newborn hearing screening protocol. *Pediatrics, 116*, 663–672.

Joint Committee on Infant Hearing. (1982, December). Joint Committee on Infant Hearing 1982 position statement. *Asha, 24*(12), 1017–1018. Available from www.jcih.org

Joint Committee on Infant Hearing. (1991). Joint Committee on Infant Hearing 1990 position statement. *Asha, 33*(3), 3–6. Available from www.jcih.org

Joint Committee on Infant Hearing. (1994). Joint Committee on Infant Hearing: 1994 position statement. *Asha, 36*(12), 38–41. Available from www.jcih.org

Joint Committee on Infant Hearing. (2000). Year 2000 Position Statement: Principles and guidelines for early hearing detection and intervention programs. *American Journal of Audiology, 9*, 9–29. Available from www.jcih.org

Joint Committee on Infant Hearing. (2007). Year 2007 position statement: Principles and guidelines for early hearing detection and intervention programs. *Pediatrics, 120*, 898–921. Available from www.asha .org/policy

Kennedy, M. B., McCann, D. C., Campbell, M. J., Law, C. M., Mellee, M., Petrou, S., et al. (2006). Language ability after early detection of permanent childhood hearing impairment. *New England Journal of Medicine, 354*, 2131–2141.

Lederberg, A., & Golbach, T. (2002). Parenting stress and social support in hearing mothers of deaf and hearing children: A longitudinal study. *Journal of Deaf Studies and Deaf Education, 7,* 330–345.

Luterman, D. (1999). *The young deaf child.* Baltimore, MD: York Press.

Luterman, D. M. (2001). *Counseling persons with communication disorders and their families* (4th ed.). Austin, TX: Pro-Ed.

Luterman, D. (2006a). Children with hearing loss: A family guide. *Hearing Review, 13*(11), 18–24.

Luterman, D. (2006b, March 21). The counseling relationship. *The ASHA Leader, 11*(4), 8–9. Available from www.asha.org/Publications/leader/2006/060321/f060321b/

Luterman, D. (2007, May 8). Technology and early childhood deafness. *The ASHA Leader, 12*(6), 43. Available from www.asha.org/Publications/leader/2007/070508/070508g/

Luterman, D., & Kurtzer-White, E. (1999). Identifying hearing loss: Parents' needs. *American Journal of Audiology, 8,* 13–18.

Martin, F. N., Barr, M. M., & Bernstein, M. (1992). Professional attitudes regarding counseling of hearing-impaired adults. *American Journal of Otology, 13,* 279–287.

Martin, F. N., Krall, L., & O'Neal, J. (1989). The diagnosis of acquired hearing loss: Patient reactions. *Asha, 31*(11), 47–50.

Matkin, N. (1988). Key considerations in counseling parents of hearing-impaired children. *Seminars in Speech and Language, 9*(3), 209–222.

Matkin, N. (1998). The challenge of providing family-centered services. In F. Bess (Ed.), *Children with hearing impairment: Contemporary trends* (pp. 299–304). Nashville, TN: Vanderbilt Bill Wilkerson Center Press.

Mavrolas, C. (1990). *Attachment behavior of hearing-impaired infants and their hearing mothers: Maternal and infant contributions.* (Unpublished doctoral dissertation.) Northwestern University, Evanston, IL

McCarthy, P., Culpepper, N. B., & Lucks, L. (1986). Variability in counseling experiences and training among ESB-accredited programs. *Asha, 28*(9), 49–52.

Meadow-Orlans, K. (1995). Sources of stress for mothers and fathers of deaf and hard of hearing infants. *American Annals of the Deaf, 140,* 352–357.

Moeller, M. P. (2000). Early intervention and language development in children who are deaf and hard of hearing. *Pediatrics, 106*(3), E43. Retrieved from www.pediatrics.org/cgi/content/full/106/3/e43

National Center for Hearing Assessment and Management. (2007). *EHDI legislation.* Available from www.infanthearing.org/legislative/index.html

National Institutes of Health. (1993). *Early identification of hearing impairment in infants and young children.* NIH Consensus Development Conference Statement. Retrieved from http://consensus.nih.gov/1993/1993HearingInfantsChildren092html.htm

Prior, M., Glazner, J., Sanson, A., & Debelle, G. (1988). Research note: Temperament and behavioral adjustment in hearing impaired children. *Journal of Child Psychology and Psychiatry, 29,* 209–216.

Radke-Yarrow, M. (1998). *Children of depressed mothers: From early childhood to maturity.* New York, NY: Cambridge University Press.

Scorgie, K., Wilgosh, L., & McDonald, L. (1998). Stress and coping in families of children with disabilities: An examination of recent literature. *Developmental Disabilities Bulletin, 26,* 22–42.

Scott, D. M. (2002). Multicultural aspects of hearing disorders and audiology. In D. E. Battle (Ed.), *Communication disorders in multicultural populations* (pp. 335–360). Woburn, MA: Butterworth-Heinemann.

Tharpe, A. M., & Clayton, E. W. (1997). Newborn hearing screening: Issues in legal liability and quality assurance. *American Journal of Audiology, 6*(2), 5–12.

U.S. Department of Health and Human Services, Public Health Service. (1990). *Healthy People 2000: National health promotion and disease prevention objectives for the nation* (DHHS Publication No. [PHS] 91-50212). Washington, DC: U.S. Government Printing Office.

Watkin, P. M., Beckman, A., & Baldwin, M. (1995). The views of parents of hearing impaired children on the need for neonatal screening. *British Journal of Audiology, 29,* 259–262.

Watson, S. M., Henggeler, S. W., & Whelan, J. P. (1990). Family functioning and the social adaptation of hearing-impaired youths. *Journal of Abnormal Child Psychology, 18,* 143–163.

Webster-Stratton, C. (1990). Stress: A potential disrupter of parent perceptions and family interactions. *Journal of Clinical Child Psychology, 19,* 302–312.

Yoshinaga-Itano, C., Sedey, A. L., Coulter, D. K., & Mehl, A. L. (1998). Language of early- and later-identified children with hearing loss. *Pediatrics, 102,* 1161–1171.

Young, A., & Tattersall, H. (2007). Universal newborn hearing screening and early identification of deafness: Parents' responses to knowing early and their expectations of child communication development. *Journal of Deaf Studies and Deaf Education, 12*(2), 209–220.

Index

Note: Page numbers in **bold** reference non-text material.